Feeding Horses

This concise handbook provides evidence-based, practical horse nutrition accessible to all readers. Standing out from very dense, theoretical and practical horse nutrition books, it arms equine students, veterinary students and horse owners with practically applicable information, bringing theory and practice together.

At the end of each chapter, veterinarian and equine nutrition experts Dr Gulsah Kaya Karasu and Dr Peter Huntington provide guidance on practical applications, calculations and the real-life use of information. For example, how is gastric ulcer formation triggered by traditional horse feeding? How can the risk of gastric ulcer formation be reduced with evidence-based feeding?

Divided into four parts, the book covers the horse's digestive system, types of feeds, formulating rations, and nutrition-related health disorders. Its scientifically validated, practical information will be invaluable for horse owners, students and trainers, equine nutritionists and practitioners within the equine industry.

Feeding Horses

An Evidence-Based Approach to Equine Nutrition

Dr. Gulsah Kaya Karasu
Dr. Peter Huntington

CRC Press
Taylor & Francis Group
Boca Raton London New York

CRC Press is an imprint of the
Taylor & Francis Group, an **informa** business

Designed Cover Image: ShutterStock ID: 429204064

First edition published 2025
by CRC Press
2385 NW Executive Center Drive, Suite 320, Boca Raton FL 33431

and by CRC Press
4 Park Square, Milton Park, Abingdon, Oxon, OX14 4RN

CRC Press is an imprint of Taylor & Francis Group, LLC

ISBN: 9781032459394 (hbk)
ISBN: 9781032459257 (pbk)
ISBN: 9781003379355 (ebk)

DOI: 10.1201/9781003379355

Typeset in Sabon
by Deanta Global Publishing Services, Chennai, India

Contents

Acknowledgement

We would like to thank Prof. Dr Christine Iben, a retired professor from the University of Veterinary Medicine Vienna, Austria, for her invaluable guidance on this book. We extend our sincere appreciation to our esteemed nutritional mentors: Dr Pat Harris, Head of Equine Research at the WALTHAM Centre for Pet Nutrition and Director of Science for MARS Horsecare; Dr Joe Pagan of Kentucky Equine Research; and Dr Steve Jackson of Bluegrass Equine Nutrition. Their wealth of knowledge, insights, and encouragement have been instrumental in shaping our approach to equine nutrition and enhancing the content of this book.

The authors

Gulsah Kaya Karasu began her veterinary medicine career at Istanbul University Veterinary Medicine, where her passion for horses was sparked during an internship at Liverpool University Leahurst Equine Hospital in the United Kingdom, from which she graduated in 2004. Driven by this early dedication, she earned her doctorate in 2009 from Vienna Veterinary University in Austria, focusing on "colic risk factors in horses." Her outstanding thesis earned her the prestigious Von Fircks Stipendium at the university, which subsequently opened up new opportunities in her career. Gulsah's career then took her around the world, including fellowships at Blue Ridge Equine Hospital in the US. In 2011, she was appointed as an associate professor at Istanbul Aydın University and pursued further education in equine medicine at Liverpool University. Her commitment to equine health led her to follow the European College of Veterinary and Comparative Nutrition Residency (ECVCN) program. She also served as a clinical nutrition advisor and practitioner at the Turkish Jockey Club Racecourse Equine Hospital. She has done technical consulting for major horse-feed companies and farms, and her insightful articles have appeared in a number of equine magazines. She currently lives in the Netherlands and works as a senior lecturer and researcher at Van Hall Larenstein University's equine department. She also founded AGG Equine Nutrition Consultancy, which offers international consulting services.

Peter Huntington's interest in horses was sparked by spending school holidays with his uncle John Williams who is a farmer and cowboy. He graduated from the University of Melbourne Veterinary faculty with honors in 1981, before spending time working in private practice and as an equine specialist for the Victorian Department of Agriculture, gaining a membership of the Australian College of Veterinary Scientists. He has worked in equine nutrition since 1993 and has been director of nutrition for Kentucky Equine Research Australasia since 1998. In that time, he has consulted horse owners, breeders, trainers, feed companies, and veterinarians in many countries, as well as lectured and written on equine nutrition and feeding for many audiences. He is the author of the best-seller *Horse Sense – The Australian and New Zealand Guide to Horse Husbandry.*

List of abbreviations

Units of measurement (explanation)

Kilogram: kg (Metric unit of mass; equivalent to 1000 grams)
Gram: g (Metric unit of mass)
Milligram: mg (Metric unit of mass; one-thousandth of a gram)
Liter: L (Metric unit of volume)
Milliliter: mL (Metric unit of volume; one-thousandth of a liter)
Meter: m (Metric unit of length)

Energy units

Kilocalorie: kcal (Unit of energy; equivalent to 1000 calories)
Megacalorie: Mcal (Unit of energy; equivalent to one million calories)
Megajoule: MJ (Unit of energy; equivalent to one million joules)

Small-quantity units

Microgram: µg (Metric unit of mass; one-millionth of a gram)

Concentration units

Parts per million: ppm (Unit of concentration; one part in a million parts)
Milligrams per kilogram: mg/kg
Parts per million (ppm) per kilogram: ppm/kg
Grams per kilogram: g/kg
International unit: IU (Unit of measurement for the amount of a fat soluble vitamin expressed as IU/kg)

Introduction

Nutrition is essential to the well-being and long-term health of horses, with their dietary needs evolving through various life stages. The goal of this book is to educate readers about equine digestion, feeds, basic ration calculation, and the profound influence of nutrition on horses' overall health and vitality. The book thus attempts to provide accurate information that will help horse owners, riders, and managers understand the foundational principles of equine nutrition, referencing numerous publications to establish a basis in scientific data. It discusses feeding management principles that distinguish horses from other domesticated animals, highlighting their distinctive nature as herbivores with small stomachs and unique digestive tracts. The importance of understanding the equine digestive tract is highlighted throughout the book to emphasize its critical role in horse health.

In addition, the book explores common feed sources, digestion, and the impact of nutrients on horse health, relying on literature to provide comprehensive insights. It emphasizes the individuality of horses and challenges the notion of a generic approach to equine diets, urging caregivers to tailor feeding plans to each horse's unique needs.

This book's wealth of scientifically proven principles should appeal to a wide range of readers, including undergraduate animal science or equine science students, horse owners, and equine professionals.

CHAPTER 1

Understanding the equine digestive system

Knowing the science behind a horse's digestive processes will help you feed your horse better, protect its health and welfare, and understand and differentiate between fact and opinion in market advertisements for commercial horse feedstuffs and evidence-based nutrition.

Healthy diets can improve a horse's health and performance in the short and long term.

The gastrointestinal system plays more than just a crucial role in the digestion and absorption of nutrients within the bodies of animals. Within this complex system, there exists a vital component known as microbiota, which refers to the diverse community of microorganisms residing in the digestive tract of animals. These microorganisms, including bacteria, viruses, fungi, and other microbiota, have a profound influence on various aspects of an animal's health and physiology. The microbiota is a dynamic and intricate ecosystem within an animal's gastrointestinal system, with wide-ranging effects on the host's health, nutrition, immunity, and even behavior. The health status of horses is directly influenced by the structure and function of their gastrointestinal tract microbiota. By understanding the anatomy of digestion, you can make more informed decisions regarding feeding and adjust your horse's nutritional plan accordingly. Horses are categorized as non-ruminant herbivores, specifically as monogastric hindgut fermenters, meaning that the main site of microbial activity is in the large intestine of the gastrointestinal tract. Gut health encompasses various dietary aspects, such as the structure and function of the gastrointestinal barrier, the microbial composition of the gut (microbiota), and the digestion and absorption of nutrients.

DOI: 10.1201/9781003379355-1

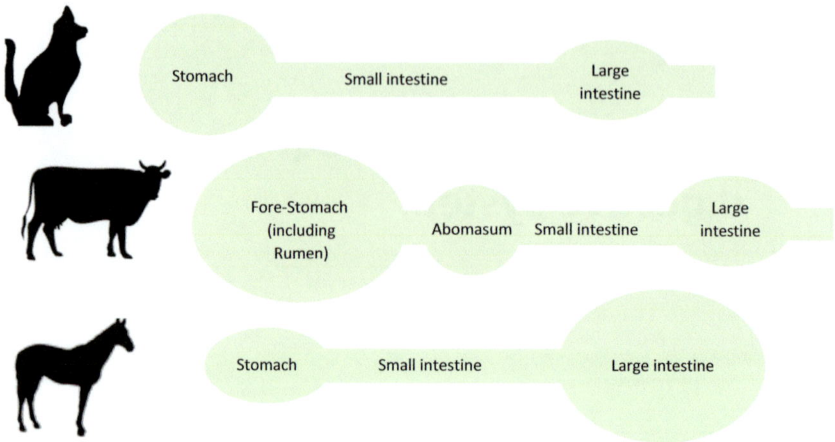

Figure 1.1 The schematic illustration of the digestive system in different animal species. Carnivores have a large stomach and a relatively short digestive tract. Ruminants are known as foregut fermenters, with the primary fermentation process taking place in their fore-stomach. Horses are hindgut fermenters, with the primary fermentation process taking place in their large intestine.

The digestive system can be divided into two main sections: the foregut and the hindgut. The foregut comprises the mouth, esophagus, stomach, and small intestine, while the hindgut consists of the cecum, colon (including the small and large colon), and rectum, and terminates at the anus. In the horse, the stomach accounts for approximately 8–10% of total digestive tract capacity (Nickel et al., 1979), while the small intestine and hindgut account for 30% and 60%, respectively (Greet, 2020; Argenzio, 1993), as illustrated in Figure 1.1.

The digestive process of horses encompasses several stages, including biting, chewing, swallowing, mixing, digestion, absorption of nutrients, and elimination of undigested material. The majority of the digesta remains in the stomach for a relatively short period, typically ranging from 2 to 6 hours. The passage through the stomach and small intestine takes approximately 2–5 hours, while the cecum and colon exhibit a longer retention time of about 35 hours (Van Weyenberg et al., 2006). Horses have evolved their digestive systems to efficiently process high-fiber forage diets. As non-ruminant herbivores, horses have adapted to consuming diets that are high in fiber and low in starch, necessitating regular daily foraging (Maisonpierre et al., 2019). Horses spend a considerable amount of time, up to 18 hours per day, engaging in foraging activities, and typically do not go without food for more than 2 to 4 hours at a time.

Horses use a combination of enzymatic digestion in the stomach and small intestine, primarily targeting soluble carbohydrates, fats, and proteins, as well as microbial fermentation of fiber in the hindgut to acquire essential nutrients. Digestion refers to the process of preparing food for absorption into the bloodstream from the gastrointestinal system while eliminating the unabsorbed residue from the body. This process involves four distinct actions:

1. **Mechanical action:** This is a purely physical process that does not alter the chemical composition of the food. It includes mastication (chewing) and tongue movements that break down food into smaller pieces and mix it with saliva (Figure 1.2). Chewing also moistens the food, facilitating easier chewing and swallowing.
2. **Secretory action:** Involves the secretion of digestive juices by salivary glands, stomach, liver, and pancreas. These digestive juices aid in breaking down complex food substances into simpler components.
3. **Chemical action:** Occurs when stomach chemicals break down complex molecules like proteins, fats, and carbohydrates into smaller fragments.
4. **Microbial action:** Involves the breakdown of food through the fermentation process, aided by billions of naturally occurring microbes, such as bacteria and protozoa.

By applying these combined actions, horses efficiently extract nutrients from their diet to use in their bodies. The digestive process of energy sources in horses is not uniform and can vary depending on the specific feed components they consume. This variability is depicted in Table 1.1, where you can find information on the common sources of feed for horses and the resultant end products of digestion. This table serves as a valuable resource for understanding how different dietary elements are processed within a horse's digestive system, highlighting the diverse pathways and final outcomes that are dependent on the specific nutrients they ingest.

You will gain a better understanding of why horses require a specific nutrition plan as you learn about the function and anatomy of the various digestive tract components.

1.1 Foregut anatomy and digestion

Mouth

The first segment of the digestive tract is the mouth, encompassing various structures such as the tongue, teeth, lips, mouth cavity, gums, salivary glands, vestibule, and the hard and soft palates. Horses typically possess 24 cheek teeth, with three premolars and three molars present in each quadrant. When consuming feed, horses employ their lips and teeth. Among these structures, the upper lip holds significant importance as it is sensitive, sturdy, and capable of mobility, enabling it to effectively grasp food.

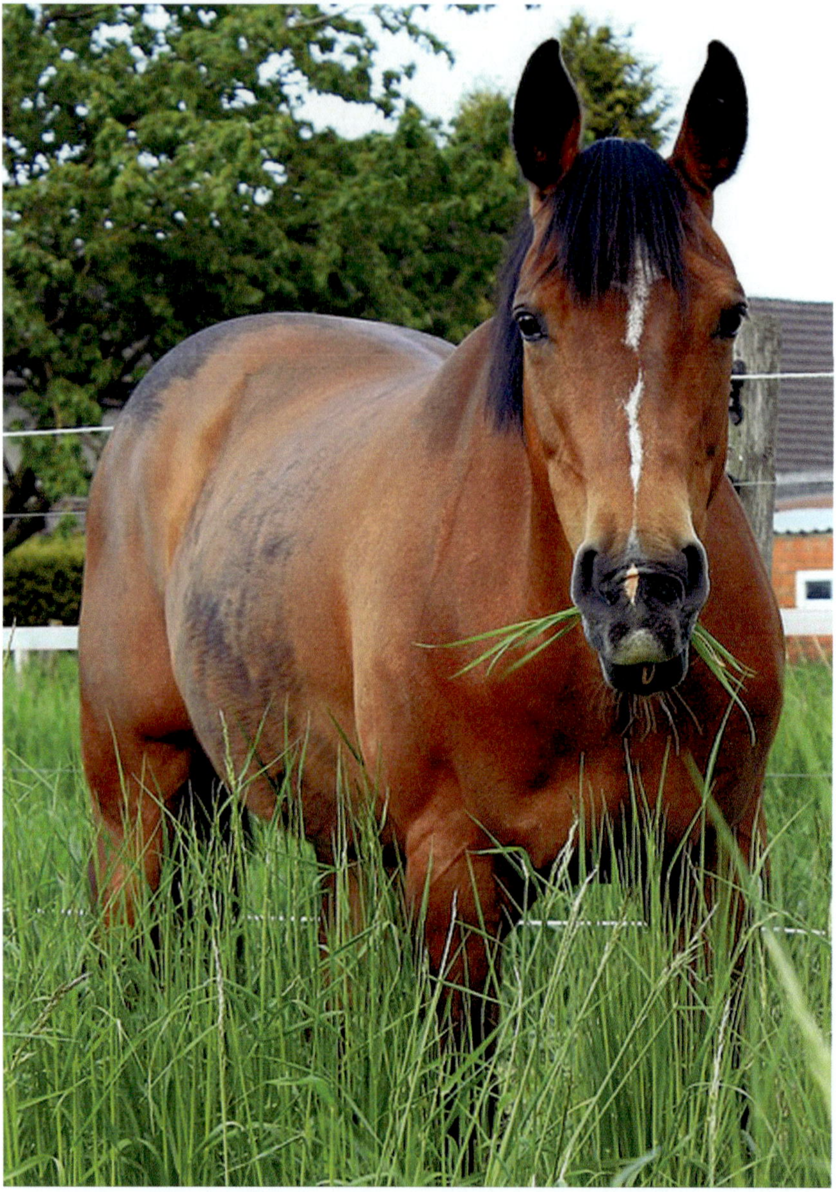

Figure 1.2 Horse chewing grass.

During grazing, the upper lip pushes grass between the upper and lower incisors, which are responsible for cutting it. The tongue then moves the food toward the molars located at the back of the mouth for grinding. In cases where horses are fed loose feed from a feeder, the tongue collaborates with the lips to collect the feed. The molars play a crucial role in grinding food, reducing its particle size (Frape, 2004).

Table 1.1 The main feed constituents, their common sources, the method, and end products of digestion

Energy source	*Fiber*	*Starch and sugar*		*Fat*	*Protein*
Common feed source	Hay, Haylage, sugar beet pulp Grass	Oats, barley, maize, molasses, grass Fructans in Grasses		Vegetable oil	Soyabean meal, canola meal
Site of absorption	Large intestine	Preferred Small intestine	Undigested starch or fructan sugars Large intestine	Small intestine	Small intestine
Method of digestion	Fermentation	Enzymatic digestion	Fermentation	Enzymatic digestion	Enzymatic digestion
End-product of digestion	Volatile fatty acids (VFA) (acetate, propionate, butyrate)	Sugars	Lactic acid and VFA (acetate, propionate, butyrate)	Fatty acids; glycerol	Amino acids

Source: adapted from Bishop, 2005

The process of mastication, or chewing, involves the intricate coordination of jaw movements, saliva secretion, and food mixing with the tongue (Bonin et al., 2007). Mastication plays a vital role in crushing and thoroughly mixing food with saliva to form a bolus that can be easily swallowed. Horses produce saliva exclusively during chewing, and it is secreted by three salivary glands: the parotid, mandibular (submandibular), and sublingual glands, named based on their anatomical location. Saliva serves the dual purpose of moistening food (lubrication) and acting as a gastric buffer, initiating the digestive process (Alexander, 1966). Equine saliva consists primarily of over 99% water, along with components like mucus, bicarbonate, sodium, potassium, chloride ions, phosphorus (P), lactate, cholesterol, fatty acids, glucose, hormones (e.g., cortisol), triglycerides, urea, and uric acid (Lindner et al., 2000). Although saliva contains small amounts of the enzyme amylase, which aids in starch digestion by breaking it down into smaller molecules, horses have relatively low concentrations of amylase compared to humans. On average, horses have reported amylase concentrations of 0.44 U/mL, while humans have an average of 77 U/mL (Varloud, 2006).

In horses, the intake of food and the act of mastication have a direct impact on the rate of salivary secretion. An adult horse has the capacity to produce approximately 35–40 liters of saliva per day, with a pH ranging from 8.6 to 9.1 (Meyer, 1985; Moeller et al., 2008). The amount of saliva secreted is influenced by both the physical composition of the meal and the time required for thorough mastication (Meyer, 1985; Meyer et al., 1986). Notable examples provide a better understanding of this relationship, as consumption of hay leads to at least three times more saliva production than with concentrate feed, as shown in Table 1.2 (Meyer et al., 1986).

The chewing behavior of horses is influenced by various factors, including the physical characteristics of the feed and the size of the meal. Different feeds, such as concentrates and roughages, lead to distinct chewing patterns in horses (Bochnia et al., 2017). Horses typically make 800 to 1200 chewing movements per kilogram of concentrate, whereas forage requires 3000 to 3500 chewing movements per kilogram. Forage necessitates more extensive jaw sweeps compared to concentrates. The particles of hay found

Table 1.2 Correlation between equine feed intake and saliva production

Feed sources (as fed 1 kg)	*Saliva production (liters) by horse*
Hay	5.8
Straw	5.2
Fresh grass	0.59
Pellet compound feed	1.7

Source: Meyer et al., 1986

in the stomach of a horse with normal teeth are typically very small, often less than 1 mm in size (Meyer et al., 1975). Since mastication stimulates saliva production, horses tend to secrete less saliva when fed concentrates than when fed roughage (Frape, 2004).

The type of forage consumed by horses has no significant impact on the concentrations of salivary electrolytes such as potassium, calcium, bicarbonate, and phosphate (Lundström et al., 2020). However, when it comes to pelleted feed with a length of around 16.5 mm, horses ingest it at a significantly faster rate and chew it more frequently compared to crushed oat grains or muesli feeds (Bochnia et al., 2017). Increased speed in consuming feed can lead to adverse effects, such as the risk of choking, reduced saliva production, and elevated stomach acidity. This risk is further heightened when horses consume feed with a high starch content, making them more susceptible to developing gastric ulcers. Therefore, prolonged fasting periods and high-concentrate diets can decrease saliva production and potentially harm the health of the horse's stomach.

Esophagus

The generation of significant amounts of saliva facilitates the movement of feed through the approximately 1.2–1.5 m esophagus and provides buffering properties to the digested material (Cunha, 1991). The horse's esophagus is a critical component of its digestive system, serving as a muscular conduit that links the pharynx to the stomach (Figure 1.3). Its primary role is to facilitate the smooth passage of food, or bolus, from the mouth to the stomach. This process is orchestrated by rhythmic contractions of the esophageal muscles, known as peristalsis, which propel the ingested material downward. The act of swallowing, scientifically referred to as deglutition, involves a complex sequence of movements, transporting food seamlessly from the mouth through the pharynx and esophagus to the stomach (Frape, 2004; Dicks et al., 2014).

How can saliva be used as a non-invasive diagnostic taste sample in horses?

The composition of saliva can be affected by systemic diseases. There has been growing interest in utilizing saliva as a diagnostic fluid, primarily due to its ease of collection through non-invasive procedures. In recent years, the term "sialochemistry," which originated in human medicine, has also been adopted for use in the context of horses, as demonstrated by the following examples.

- In horses, non-invasive biomarkers such as salivary-glutamyl transferase, salivary alpha-amylase (sAA), creatine kinase (CK), urea, total bilirubin, certain proteins, and phosphorus levels can be elevated and serve as indicators for acute abdominal diseases (Contreras-Aguilar et al., 2019) or gastric ulcers (Muñoz-Prieto et al., 2023).

- A recent advancement in equine diagnostics involves the creation of a convenient saliva test for detecting tapeworm infections in horses and evaluating its efficacy in guiding anthelmintic treatment. This innovative diagnostic method has the potential to reduce the reliance on anthelmintic treatments (Lightbody et al., 2018).

Can a horse vomit?

Horses cannot vomit due to the one-way peristaltic movement in horses from the pharynx to the stomach. The act of regurgitation presents a time of notable risk to horses, potentially coinciding with or resulting in the rupture of their stomach or pneumonia, where the regurgitated material may enter the lungs, causing inflammation and infection in one or both lungs.

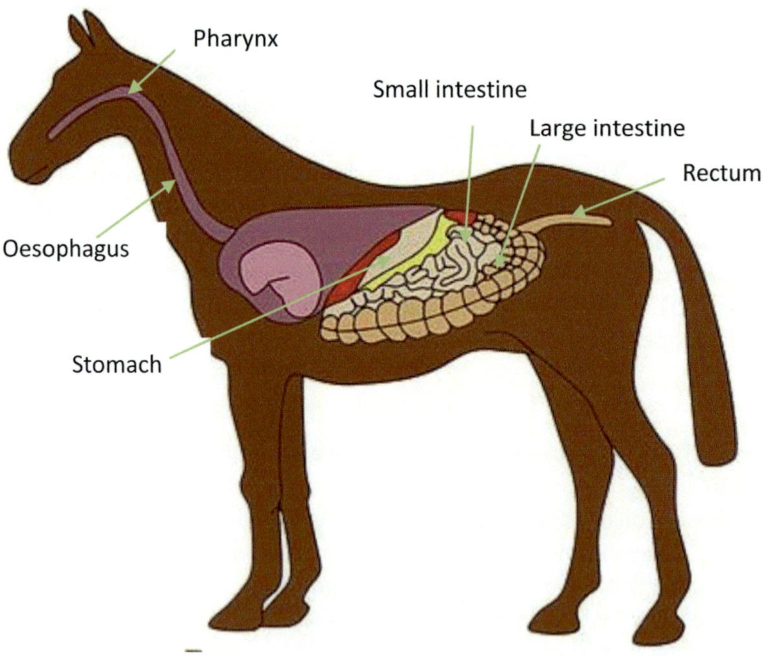

Figure 1.3 Equine digestive system. Photo by Kowalska-Art/iStockphoto.com.

Stomach

As equine saliva has no digestive enzyme activity (Al Jassim & Andrews, 2009), unlike in other species, the stomach is the first site of digestion. Understanding the anatomy and digestion of the equine stomach is thus critical for healthy horse feeding practices and the prevention of gastrointestinal tract diseases in horses.

The stomach of a horse is distinguished by certain characteristics. The stomach accounts for approximately 8% of horses' total digestive tract capacity. A 500-kg adult horse's stomach has a capacity of 8 to 15 liters (Nickel et al., 1979). This implies that a horse's stomach is approximately one to two times the size of a standard basketball, given that a standard basketball typically has a volume ranging from 7.5 to 8.5 liters. The horse has proportionally the smallest stomach among domesticated animals (Figure 1.1). The stomach is divided into two sections: the top, known as the squamous region, and the bottom, known as the glandular region, separated by a distinct line known as the margo plicatus (Figure 1.4).

The squamous region of the stomach is pale yellow to white in color and has a smooth, gleaming surface (Hewetson & Tallon, 2021). This region of the stomach does not produce digestive juices, has no absorptive capacity, no defense against gastric acid, and functions solely as a protective barrier.

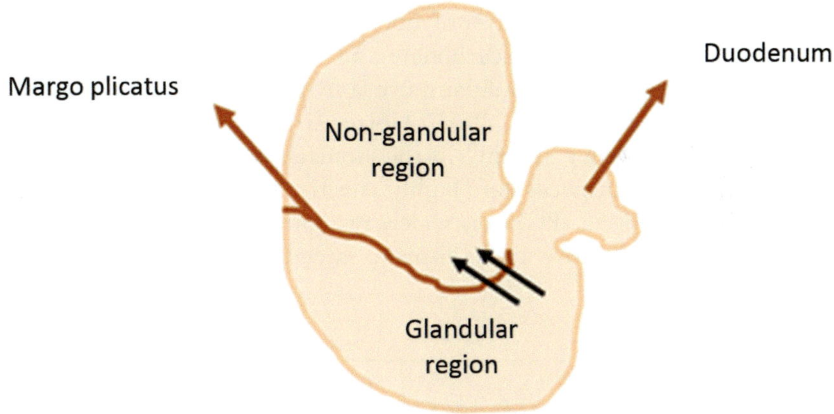

Figure 1.4 A schematic illustration of the stomach of a horse. The upper portion of the stomach is lined with non-glandular squamous cells and lacks a protective mechanism, whereas the lower portion is lined with glandular cells and has its own protective mechanism. The black arrows represent the proposed mechanism by which exercise causes a change in pH (acidity) in the upper portion of the stomach by compressing the abdominal muscles more than at rest, especially if the stomach is empty. This increased acidity can result in gastric ulcers in the squamous region of the stomach.

The glandular region consists of mucus-producing cells and gastric glands, and secretes hydrochloric acid, pepsin, bicarbonate, and mucus. The cardiac, fundic, and pyloric portions of the stomach are all parts of the glandular region (Merritt & Julliand, 2013).

- **The cardiac region:** This region is small, and unfortunately there is little knowledge of it; it may have a high pH environment due to saliva flow, limited exposure to gastric acid, and anaerobic gram-positive microbial colonization.
- **The fundic region:** This region secretes mucus, gastric acids, hydrochloric acid (HCl), and digestive enzymes such as pepsinogen and lipase (Greet, 2020). The parietal cells of the fundic mucosa release HCl and intrinsic factors. Hydrochloric acid is the primary secretory product of the horse's stomach, as it is in all species (Baker & Gerring, 1993). The horse's stomach continuously secretes variable amounts of HCl, and acid secretion occurs even when the horse is fasting, which is known as basal secretion. The secretion of HCl into the stomach induces an acidic gastric environment (pH 2–5) (Husted et al., 2008).
- **The pyloric region:** This region secretes gastric acid and gastric juice continuously, even when fasting (Greet, 2020).

The glandular mucosa in the horse's stomach has its own protective mechanism, which includes a thick layer of mucus, robust blood flow, and the natural production of sodium bicarbonate and mucus. These elements work together to safeguard the glandular mucosa from damage caused by gastric acid (Flemström & Isenberg, 2001). Holzer (1998) proposed the concept of a "neural emergency system" in the stomach, where receptors within the gastric glandular mucosa are highly sensitive to the presence of gastric acid. Prostaglandin-E2 (PGE2) is widely recognized as one of the key factors that induce protective mechanisms to safeguard the glandular mucosa (Holzer, 1998).

What is gastric juice?

Gastric juice in horses is composed of a unique mixture of water, mucus, pepsin, HCl, intrinsic factor for vitamin B12 absorption, somatostatin, and inorganic salts. Horses produce an estimated 10 to 30 liters of gastric juice per day. It is believed that gastric juice secretion in the horse's stomach is continuous, but it increases when food is present. Within the stomach, the food material and saliva combines with gastric juice to form chyme. Subsequently, the chyme is released into the first part of the small intestine, known as the duodenum.

What is the normal pH range for a horse's stomach?

The stomach's pH levels vary throughout different regions, ranging from slightly basic (pH 6–7) near the esophagus to highly acidic (pH 1–2) near the duodenum. When horses eat, the density of the feed affects its positioning in the stomach. Low-density feed remains near the top, mixing with saliva to maintain a closer-to-neutral pH (around pH 7). Higher-density feed settles lower, entering the glandular portion of the stomach, which has the lowest pH due to hydrochloric acid secretion by parietal cells (Merritt, 2003). The glandular section is protected by mucus, while the squamous upper part lacks this protection. Horses tend to consume a significant portion of their roughage during the daytime (Ellis et al., 2015), and the presence of fibrous ingesta in the stomach aids in maintaining a normal pH of gastric content. This fibrous material also facilitates acid buffering in the squamous area of the stomach. Due to the considerably higher pH levels observed in the squamous stomach of horses during the day, which can persist for up to 5 hours after feeding (Husted et al., 2008), it is crucial to feed horses frequently and avoid intervals longer than 6 hours to reduce the risk of equine gastric ulcers.

In neonatal foals, the pH in the proximal and distal stomach exhibits significant variability, with an average pH of 5.5 (Wise et al., 2020). At birth, the squamous mucosa is relatively thin and gradually thickens as the foal matures, potentially due to increased exposure to gastric acid (Murray & Mahaffey, 1993).

The role of the stomach in digestion and absorption in horses

The stomach has essential roles in the digestive process, including the mixing, storage, and release of feed into the small intestine. It actively participates in digestion by initiating the pre-digestion of proteins and fats, as well as physically breaking down the feed before it enters the small intestine, where the absorption of nutrients takes place. The stomach utilizes HCl and enzymes like pepsin to facilitate the processes of digestion and fermentation.

Enzymatic digestion in the horse's stomach

The equine stomach, like in other mammals, produces two main digestive enzymes: pepsin and gastric lipase. However, the specific roles of pepsin and lipase in equine digestion are not well understood, as indicated by the lack of available information (Merritt & Julliand, 2013).

- Pepsinogen is the primary secretion of the zymogen (chief) cells located in the glands of the fundic and pyloric regions of the equine stomach. It undergoes conversion to pepsin when the pH of the surrounding medium reaches 4.0. The digestion of proteins is facilitated by the combination of HCl. However, the relatively brief transit time of ingested material within the stomach results in a limited extent of complete protein digestion; nevertheless, this initial phase of protein breakdown serves as a vital starting point in the overall protein digestion process.

- Gastric lipase, produced by the zymogen cells in the glands of the fundic region, is also present in significant amounts in horses. It has an optimal pH range between 4.0 and 6.0. Gastric lipase is likely involved in the partial digestion of feed fats triacylglycerols (TAG), breaking them down into diacylglycerols and free fatty acids.

Fermentation in the horse's stomach

The fermentation capacity of the stomach microbiota in equine nutrition is often overlooked, and there is limited knowledge regarding the diversity and structure of bacteria in the equine stomach. However, studies have indicated a high concentration of total anaerobes on the mucosa of the squamous and glandular cardiac regions in the empty stomach. Previous research has identified the presence of microflora in the equine stomach, with *Lactobacillus* spp., *Streptococcus* spp., and *Sarcina* spp. being the most abundant bacteria (Perkins et al., 2012; Glatter et al., 2019). Surprisingly, the acidic conditions of the stomach do not prevent the presence of a large number of bacteria (Varloud, 2006). However, despite high microbial densities, the fermentative activity of bacteria is low in the empty stomach, leading to low end-product concentrations. Bacteria in the equine stomach, including *Streptococcus bovis*, *S. equi* (*S. equinus*), *Lactobacillus salivarius*, *L. mucosae*, *L. delbrueckii*, and *Mitsuokella jalaludinii*, can utilize starch or non-structural carbohydrates from the diet as a carbon source (Varloud et al., 2007). The concentration of cellulolytic bacteria in the horse's stomach has been reported to be negligible (De Fombelle et al., 2004). Fermentation primarily occurs in the squamous part of the stomach.

In foals, different grains such as corn, oats, and barley do not significantly affect the microbial diversity of stomach content. However, the relative abundance of bacteria varies significantly in response to different diets. For instance, oats have been found to increase the relative abundance of Firmicutes, Lactobacillaceae, *Lactobacillus* spp, and *Lactobacillus hayakitensis* in foals.

The concentration of lactate-utilizing bacteria in the horse's stomach increases at 30 minutes (De Fombelle et al., 2004) and 210 minutes after a meal (Varloud et al., 2007). The gastric microflora, particularly the high proportion of amylolytic bacteria, significantly influences starch digestion. Starch is degraded into lactate and VFA in the stomach, while in the small intestine, it is converted into glucose.

This results in a decrease in the pH of the digesta to approximately 2.6 (Frape, 2010). In addition, the presence of VFAs in the stomach, particularly during periods of extended fasting or high-grain diets, can contribute to the erosion of gastric mucosa, potentially leading to equine gastric ulcer syndrome (EGUS). Exceeding suggested intake thresholds for starch and water-soluble carbohydrates, such as 1.0 g/kg body weight/meal or 2.0 g/kg body weight/day, may lead to an increased risk of gastric ulceration (Luthersson et al., 2009; Harris & Dunnett, 2018).

The physiology of gastric emptying

Gastric emptying, the process of transferring stomach contents to the duodenum, involves multiple simultaneous actions, including relaxation of the proximal stomach, suppression of antral motility, and stimulation of pyloric contraction (Lorenzo-Figueras et al., 2005). The composition of the diet plays a role in stomach digestion. The rate of gastric emptying can be influenced by factors such as the composition, volume, physical structure, energy density, and osmolarity of the meal (Meyer et al., 1986). For instance, a meal rich in starch (1.25 g starch/kg body weight) leads to slower gastric emptying compared to a meal with lower starch content (0.66 g starch/kg body weight) (Metayer et al., 2004). Forage requires thorough chewing and stimulates saliva production, which has a buffering and lubricating effect on digesta. It moves more slowly through the digestive tract, promoting efficient digestion processes (Frape, 2004; Greet, 2020) when compared to grains. In contrast, when horses consume finely chopped, pelleted particles or grains, these materials tend to pass quickly through the stomach with limited digestion (Frape, 2004). High-fat meals slow stomach emptying and lowers the glycemic and insulinemic response to a meal (Pagan, 1998). This difference in gastric transit time can have implications for nutrient absorption and overall digestive efficiency in horses, highlighting the importance of considering meal composition and particle size when formulating equine diets.

Although the stomach size is small, ingesta moves through it relatively swiftly, but a significant portion remains in the anaerobic fundic section for 2–6 hours. Ingesta refers to partially digested food in the stomach. As soon as feeding begins and fresh food enters the stomach, some of the ingesta already present will pass into the small intestine. Often, the feed consumed at the beginning of a meal may enter the small intestine before the meal is completed. The pyloric sphincter regulates the movement of food from the stomach to the small intestine.

Small intestine

In horses, like other mammals, the small intestine serves as the link between the stomach and the large intestine (Figure 1.3). In relation to the horse's body size, the small intestine is relatively short, measuring approximately 25 m in length in a 500-kg adult horse (Geor et al., 2013). It consists of three distinct sections: the duodenum, jejunum, and ileum. Shaped like an "S," it also houses the pancreas. The duodenum, which is about 1–1.5 m long, is connected to the stomach through the pylorus and receives the pancreatic and bile ducts. The jejunum and ileum are suspended from the body wall by the mesentery. The jejunum covers the largest portion of the small intestine, while the ileum is the shortest section, measuring approximately 1 m. The ileum connects the foregut to the hindgut through the lesser curvature of the cecum.

The mucosae and lumen of the duodenum, jejunum, and ileum contain a population of viable bacteria ranging from 10^6 to 10^7 per mL, with most of them exhibiting proteolytic activity (Mackie & Wilkins, 1988). The bacterial population in the upper gastrointestinal tract (GIT) is likely to vary due to both the rapid movement of content in the upper GIT and the constant introduction of environmental bacteria from feed and forage. For instance, a study conducted in the US with nine healthy adult horses revealed that while certain dominant taxa, such as Actinobacillus sp. and Lactobacillus sp. were present in all horses, their relative abundance differed significantly. The presence of abundant Proteobacteria in the upper GIT, commonly found in environmental samples, further supports the variation in bacterial composition (Ericsson et al., 2016).

The mucosa of the small intestine is composed of finger-like projections known as villi (Figure 1.5). These intestinal walls have folds or wrinkles that contain millions of villi, which in turn are covered with millions of smaller projections called microvilli. The presence of these villi greatly increases the surface area of the small intestine compared to a flat lining. This increased surface area enhances the small intestine's capacity to absorb nutrients. Within the microvilli, there are intestinal digestive enzymes that play a crucial role in the process of digestion. In horses, Brunner's glands serve a dual function of protecting the mucosa in the proximal duodenum by secreting bicarbonate and releasing digestive enzymes, including lipase or other unidentified substances (Pfeiffer & Dabareiner, 1992).

The role of the small intestine in digestion and absorption in horses

The small intestine is the main location for the digestion and absorption of soluble carbohydrates such as sugars and starch, proteins, lipids, fats, soluble vitamins (A, D, E, and K), and minerals. The hydrolysis of dietary non-structural carbohydrates, proteins, and fats occurs through the action of pancreatic and intestinal brush-border enzymes, especially in the presence of bile salts.

Two main factors influence digestion in the small intestine:

1. Movements of the intestinal wall
2. Secretions of pancreatic juice, bile, and intestinal juice

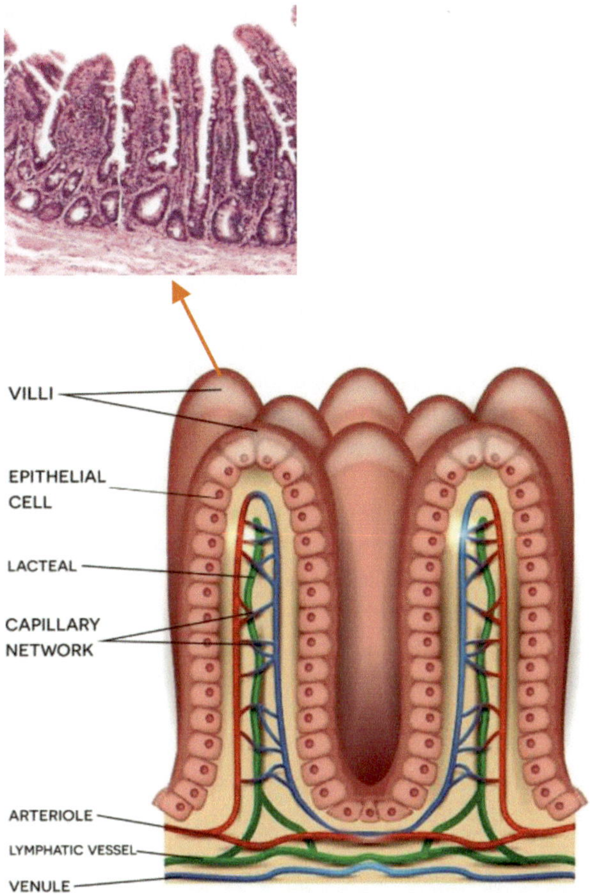

Figure 1.5 The structure of intestinal villi along with a microscopic view. Villi are finger-shaped structures found along the inner lining of the small intestine which increase the available surface area for the absorption of nutrients from digested feed. Photo by iStockphoto.com. https://www.istockphoto.com/nl/vector/intestinal-villi-anatomy-gm653494152-118853693.

In order to facilitate digestion, a significant quantity of fluid and other substances is secreted into the small intestine, primarily by the liver and pancreas. The pancreatic gland produces pancreatic juice, which contains various enzymes, including trypsin, pancreatic lipase, and pancreatic amylase. However, the concentrations of these digestive enzymes, such as amylase and trypsinogen (trypsin), are relatively low in horses compared to other species (Sandberg & Flythe, 2016). Trypsin converts proteins and partially hydrolyzed proteins into peptides and amino acids, while pancreatic lipase breaks down fats into fatty acids and glycerol, and pancreatic amylase aids in the breakdown of starch into maltose. Since horses lack a gallbladder, the liver continuously produces bile and releases it into the small intestine, which is essential for fat digestion. Bile activates pancreatic lipase, assists in fat emulsification, and aids in the absorption of fatty acids.

The small intestine is the primary site where enzymatic breakdown and absorption of digested material occur. When the acidic digesta reaches the duodenum, the pH is neutralized to 7.0 or 7.4 by bile secreted from the liver, creating an alkaline environment that enables proper enzyme function and emulsification of fats (Colville & Bassert, 2008). Bicarbonate secretion plays a crucial role in two specific sites: in the duodenum, from Brunner's glands, to protect the duodenal mucosa from acidic contents from the stomach (Pfeiffer & Dabareiner, 1992), and in the distal ileum, which is believed to support the favorable environment necessary for cecal microbes involved in fermentation (Argenzio & Stevens, 1975).

The majority of enzymatic breakdown and absorption of digested material occurs in the small intestine. The fundamental digestive processes are similar to those observed in other monogastric animals, with pancreatic and intestinal brush-border enzymes hydrolyzing dietary non-structural carbohydrates and proteins (Kienzle & Radicke, 1993; Richards et al., 2004; Merritt & Julliand, 2013). Less is known about protein and fat assimilation in horses, although it is worth noting that equine pancreatic tissue contains relatively high concentrations of lipase (Lorenzo-Figueras et al., 2007). The absorption of various nutrients such as amino acids, sugars, fatty acids, minerals, and vitamins occurs in the small intestine, which is well-equipped with villi that increase the surface area and enhance absorption.

The function of pancreatic juice in digestion

The equine pancreas is a vital organ for both the digestive and endocrine systems, where it plays key roles in enzymatic digestion and hormonal regulation. Concerning enzymatic digestion, the pancreas releases a suite of digestive enzymes, including amylase, lipase, and protease, into the small intestine, primarily the duodenum. These enzymes are integral to the breakdown of dietary carbohydrates, fats, and proteins, facilitating their absorption and subsequent utilization within the horse (Roberts, 1975).

The pancreas has an endocrine function by producing insulin, a hormone of paramount importance in governing blood glucose levels. Insulin plays a particularly pivotal role as it regulates the cellular uptake and metabolism of glucose, which is central to energy metabolism. Any disruption in insulin function, often arising from factors like obesity, insulin resistance, or pancreatic dysfunction, can precipitate various health issues, including insulin dysregulation (ID), equine metabolic syndrome (EMS), or laminitis (Loos et al., 2019).

The pancreas secretes a significant quantity of pancreatic juice containing enzymes in response to stimuli mediated by vagal nerve fibers and gastric HCl in the duodenum (Frape, 2004). An average-sized adult horse produces approximately 20–25 liters of pancreatic juice per day (Kitchen et al., 2000). Interestingly, while pancreatic secretion is continuous, the rate of secretion increases by four to five times when feed is initially introduced (Frape, 2004). Equine pancreatic juice has a neutral pH, mainly due to its bicarbonate content of 30 milliequivalents per liter, and it serves as an essential buffer against gastric acid entering the duodenum (Kitchen et al., 2000). The primary enzymes found in pancreatic juice are amylase, lipase, and proteases. Pancreatic amylase breaks down starches and carbohydrates into simpler sugars, such as maltose and dextrin. Lipase is responsible for the digestion of fats or lipids. It breaks down triglycerides into glycerol and fatty acids, which can then be absorbed and used by the horse for energy and other metabolic processes. Proteases are a group of enzymes that break down proteins into smaller peptides and amino acids. In horses, trypsin and chymotrypsin are among the proteases produced in the pancreas.

The function of bile in digestion

Bile, a secretion from the liver, has several functions. It activates pancreatic lipase, aids in the emulsification of fats, and supports the absorption of fatty acids. Bile release is triggered by the presence of gastric hydrochloric acid in the duodenum. The continuous drainage of bile from the liver through the bile duct into the duodenum aids in the emulsification of fats, primarily through the action of bile salts. Bile serves to neutralize chyme and emulsify fat, containing bile salts, bile pigments, cholesterol, and salts. Bile salts, along with pancreatic bicarbonate, maintain an alkaline pH in the small intestine and prepare fats for absorption. Similar to other species, the excretion of bile salts in horses appears to depend on the integrity of the enterohepatic circulation. Emulsification increases the interface between fat and water, facilitating the hydrolysis of neutral fats into fatty acids and glycerol by the enzyme lipase. These products are readily absorbed in the small intestine (Frape, 2004). Bile salts are also absorbed from the small intestine and transported back to the liver. They play a crucial role in solubilizing the products of lipolysis by absorbing at the interface between triacylglycerol and water. Monoacylglycerols and long-chain fatty acids interact with bile salts and phospholipids, forming mixed micelles (Geor et al., 2013). This micellar solubilization allows lipolysis products to pass through the brush border of the intestinal cells and be absorbed by enterocytes (Lengsfeld et al., 2004), as well as reforming triacylglycerols for transport into the lymphatic system (Geor et al., 2013).

Is bile reflux a normal finding in horses?

Bile reflux in horses refers to the abnormal backflow of bile from the small intestine or duodenum into the stomach. It is released into the small intestine to aid in the digestion and absorption of fats from the horse's diet. However, when bile flows backward into the stomach, it can cause various digestive problems and lead to discomfort or health issues in horses, including equine glandular gastric disease (EGGD). Due to the position of the bile and primary pancreatic ducts, there is an elevated likelihood of refluxing back into the stomach, especially when the stomach is empty (Kitchen et al., 2000). Nevertheless, reflux is deemed abnormal in horses.

Carbohydrate digestion in the small intestine

The carbohydrates found in plant materials such as hay, pasture, cereal grain, and commercial grain concentrate, which form the basis of modern equine diets, are quite diverse. Non-structural carbohydrates, including sugars, disaccharides, and starches, are primarily digested in the small intestine. On the other hand, structural carbohydrates and the sugar fructans found in grasses are resistant to enzymatic digestion in the small intestine and require fermentation by bacteria in the horse's hindgut.

Dietary carbohydrates play a vital role in providing nutrition to horses and undergo a series of intricate processes for digestion and absorption, predominantly occurring in the small intestine. The process begins with the hydrolysis of starch in the intestinal lumen by pancreatic amylase. Pancreatic α-amylase breaks down starch into the disaccharide maltose. Subsequently, maltose is further digested into simple sugars, particularly glucose, by the brush-border membrane disaccharidase enzyme called maltase. Horses exhibit high maltase activity in their small intestine. However, research has shown that the levels and activity of α-amylase in the equine intestine are relatively low compared to other species (Kienzle et al., 1994). Therefore, it is likely that the initial breakdown of starch into maltose, maltotriose, and α-dextrin represents the limiting step in starch digestion for horses fed concentrate diets rich in grain (Richards et al., 2004).

Therefore, the production of α-amylase in horses is sufficient when they are fed a high proportion of forage in their diet but becomes limited when they are fed a large amount of starch. Consequently, large meals of cereal grains (>2 g of starch/kg body weight/meal) may overwhelm the digestive capacity of the small intestine, leading to rapid fermentation of undigested starch in the hindgut (Harris & Dunnett, 2018). In a 500kg horse, this equates to a >2kg meal of barley, assuming the barley is 50% starch (as

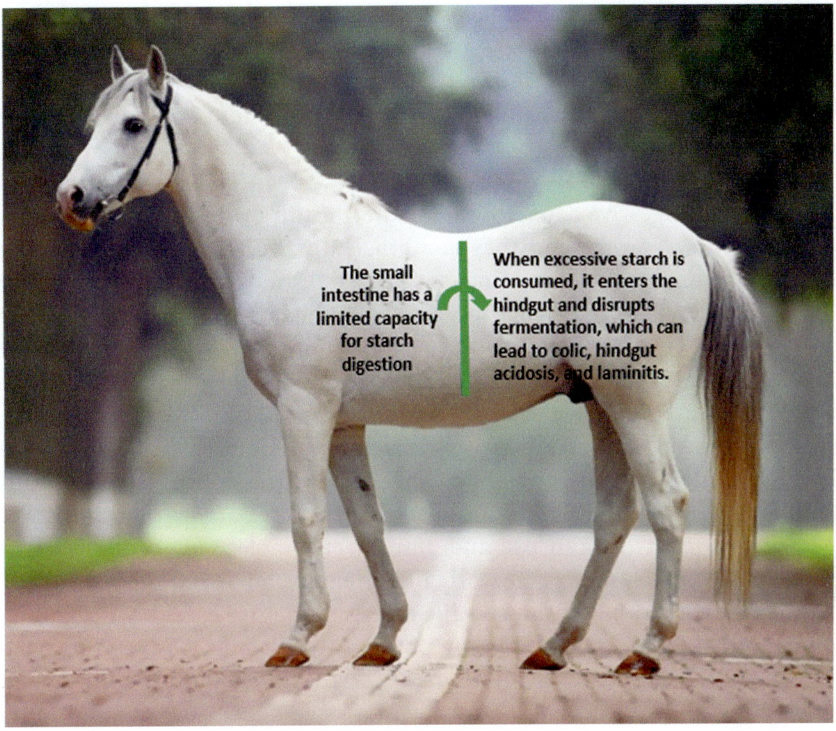
The small
intestine has a
limited capacity
for starch
digestion
When excessive starch is
consumed, it enters the
hindgut and disrupts
fermentation, which can
lead to colic, hindgut
acidosis, and laminitis.

Figure 1.6 The impact of high-starch diets on horses' health.

fed). This can potentially negatively impact gastrointestinal health, leading to the risk of conditions such as hindgut acidosis (HGA), dysbiosis, colic, and laminitis (Figure 1.6). The presence of undigested starch in the hindgut can increase the population of lactic acid-producing bacteria, which has been associated with an elevated risk of colic (Daly et al., 2012). This increased production of lactic acid and subsequent HGA can cause significant damage to the intestinal epithelium. Additionally, HGA can lead to intestinal hyperpermeability, also known as "leaky gut" (Bell et al., 2007). Horses require a longer adaptation period to enhance α-amylase activity in response to an increased high-carbohydrate diet compared to omnivorous species like pigs, and this is one of many reasons for changing feeds slowly (Richards et al., 2004).

In summary, inadequate starch digestion in the small intestine results in increased starch overflow, with digestion occurring in the large intestine, leading to hindgut disturbances and reduced nutrient absorption. When comparing two feeding regimens, one based on a high-starch diet and the other on a high-fiber diet, it was found that high levels of starch in the horse's diet were associated with an increased EGUS risk (Luthersson et al., 2009), more severe mucosal lesions in the glandular region of the stomach, as well as higher inflammation in the jejunum and pelvic flexure (Colombino et al., 2022).

Starch isn't necessarily harmful to horses, but excessive consumption beyond their digestive capacity can lead to health problems. When horses consume more starch than they can efficiently digest, it can result in an overflow of undigested starch into the large intestine and HGA, potentially disrupting the balance of microorganisms in the horse's large intestines.

Therefore, it is recommended to feed no more than 2 grams, and more recently 1 gram, of starch per kilogram of body weight per meal (Potter et al., 1992; De Fombelle et al., 2004; Julliand et al., 2006). Furthermore, starch digestion can vary depending on several factors, including intake level, botanical origin, genotype, and feed processing of cereal grains (Julliand et al., 2006). Cereal grain starch, such as oats, barley, and corn, primarily consists of amylose and amylopectin molecules. While it's true that oats are much more prececally digestible for horses compared to barley, maize (corn), and wheat, specific digestibility rates can vary depending on factors like processing and preparation (Meyer et al., 1986; Martinson et al., 2012). The apparent digestibility of cereal starch in the foregut ranges from 20% to 90%, depending on the grain and processing method, with thermal and hydrothermal processes having a greater impact than physical processes. Physical and thermal processes improve the prececal digestibility of corn and barley starch while having a minimal effect on other cereals (Julliand et al., 2006) (see Chapter 2).

After the digestion of starch, the resulting oligosaccharides undergo further hydrolysis by disaccharidases. The disaccharides, including sucrose, lactose, and maltose, are broken down into monosaccharides, specifically D-glucose, D-galactose, and D-fructose, by specific intestinal brush-border enzymes: sucrase, lactase, maltase, and β-glucosidase (Table 1.3). Here are the details:

- Sucrase and maltase, both present on the brush-border membrane of the equine small intestine (Dyer et al., 2002), are responsible for the hydrolysis of sucrose and maltose, respectively. Sucrase breaks down sucrose into glucose and fructose, while maltase hydrolyzes maltose into two molecules of glucose (Laurence & Peter, 2016). Horses possess sufficient activity of these disaccharidases in the small intestine, with sucrase activity being highest in the proximal small intestine and maltase activity distributed throughout the small intestine, including the proximal, mid, and distal sections when on a grass-based diet (Dyer et al., 2002). The jejunum and duodenum exhibit the highest sucrase

Table 1.3 Carbohydrate enzymatic digestion in the equine small intestine

Substrate	*Enzyme*	*Product*
Starch	α-amylase	Dextrins
Dextrins	a-Glucosidases	Glucose
Maltose	Maltase	Glucose and glucose
Sucrose	Sucrase	Fructose and glucose
Lactose	Lactase	Glucose and galactose

Source: adapted from Frape, 2004

and maltase activity, whereas the ileum has lower levels (Al-Rammahi, 2020).

- Lactase, which digests lactose (milk sugar), is also found in the brush-border membrane of the equine small intestine. Lactase activity is relatively low in all three regions of the small intestine, and slightly higher in the jejunum and duodenum compared to the ileum (Al-Rammahi, 2020). Lactase hydrolyzes lactose into glucose and galactose (Laurence & Peter, 2016).
- β-glucosidase, another important disaccharidase present in the intestinal juice, is referred to as neutral β-galactosidase or brush-border lactase. It plays a crucial role in the digestion of milk sugar in foals (Frape, 2004).

The mechanisms of transport for glucose and fructose are believed to be comparable in horses to those in other species. Glucose and galactose are transported across the brush-border membrane of intestinal enterocytes through the sodium-dependent glucose transporter SGLT1, whereas fructose is absorbed via the sodium-independent fructose transporter GLUT5 (Röder et al., 2014). Subsequently, these monosaccharides are transported into the systemic circulation across the basolateral membrane of the intestinal enterocyte by the sodium-independent monosaccharide transporter GLUT2 (Moran et al., 2018).

Fructans serve as storage carbohydrates and are prevalent in numerous plant species. Horses are commonly provided with cool-season grasses such as Timothy grass, Kentucky bluegrass, and ryegrass, which can accumulate fructans. Importantly, fructans do not undergo digestion in the small intestine; instead, they undergo fermentation by the microflora present in the cecum and colon. This fermentation process leads to a shift in the gut's pH levels, promoting the proliferation of gram-positive bacteria. Excessive consumption of fructans in the diet can result in an overgrowth of these gram-positive bacteria, leading to the production of endotoxins that damage the mucosal barrier and potentially leading to conditions such as laminitis.

Understanding digestion of forage in comparison with grain

Horses have evolved to thrive on continuous grazing of grass, as their digestive system is designed for the digestion of fibrous feeds in the hindgut. Within the hindgut, a large population of microorganisms facilitates the fermentation of fiber, releasing energy. This microbial fermentation produces volatile fatty acids (VFA), including acetate, propionate, and butyrate, which serve as important energy sources. These VFA are readily absorbed into the bloodstream and can be converted to glucose or fat, or utilized directly for energy. The proportions of acetate, propionate, and butyrate can vary significantly based on the diet. The composition and abundance of microorganisms in the hindgut depend on the type of diet being fed, underscoring the importance of providing sufficient fiber to maintain the health of these microorganisms.

However, it is crucial to limit the feeding of grain in horses' diets. Grain primarily consists of hydrolyzable carbohydrates, particularly starch, with a smaller portion of fiber. Horses' digestive systems are not well adapted to digest large amounts of starch, which is a complex compound composed of multiple glucose molecules bonded together. Starch digestion primarily occurs in the small intestine through the action of the enzyme amylase. If the horse's diet contains an excessive amount of starch, the small intestine may be unable to fully digest it, resulting in undigested starch reaching the hindgut. It is advisable to take care when incorporating excessive grain into a horse's diet to prevent possible health concerns, including conditions like colic and laminitis (Figure 1.6).

Protein digestion in the small intestine

Protein digestion begins in the stomach but is limited, and only a small percentage of the bacteria in the large intestine can break down proteins. This suggests that the majority of protein digestion takes place in the small intestine (Frape, 2010) (Figure 1.9). Proteins are made up of building blocks of amino acids, and during the process of protein digestion, these amino acids are produced. The small intestine contains proteolytic enzymes, also known as proteases, which break down dietary proteins into amino acids (Figure 1.7). Additionally, the pancreas secretes digestive juices into the small intestine, containing enzymes that further break down proteins into individual amino acids through the hydrolysis of peptide bonds. These amino acids are then absorbed into the bloodstream. Among the different parts of the horse's gastrointestinal tract, the ileum exhibits the highest levels of endogenous and microbial proteolytic activity compared to other areas (Kern et al., 1974). Trypsin, an enzyme, activates other oligopeptidases, including chymotrypsinogen. Pancreatic carboxypeptidases break down smaller oligopeptides into di- and tripeptides (25%) or amino acids (75%) (Johnson, 2001).

The quality of dietary protein, which refers to its amino acid composition, as well as the content and availability of crude protein, are important

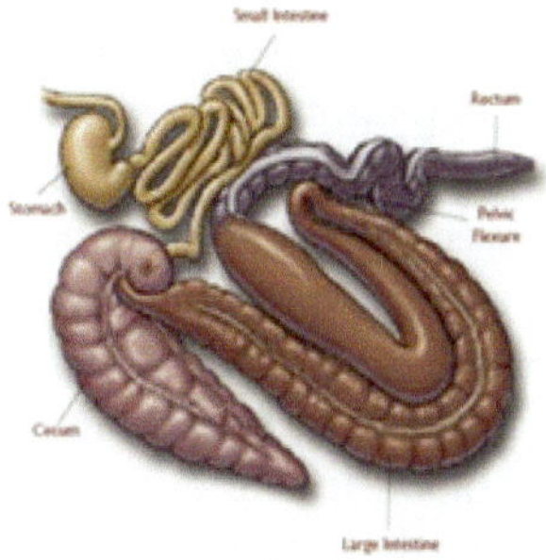

Mouth

Salivary amylase (limited amount)

Stomach

Stomach acids (chemical digestion)

Pepsin (Protein → proteoses and peptones)

Lipase (Fats → fatty acid and glycerol)

Liver

Bile salts (emulsification of lipids)

Pancreas

Amylase (Starch and dextrins → dextrins, maltose)

Lipase (Fats → fatty acids and glycerol)

Trypsin (Proteins, proteoses, polypeptides, peptones → peptones, peptides, aminoacids)

Chymotrypsin (activated by trypsin)

Small intestine

Sucrase (Sacrose → glucose + fructose)

Maltase (Maltose → glucose + glucose)

Lactase (Lactose → glucose + galactose)

Aminopeptidases (Peptides → amino acids)

Erepsin (Proteins, proteoses, polypeptides, peptones → amino acids)

Enterokinase (Trypsinogen → Trypsin)

Figure 1.7 An overview of the enzymes involved in horse digestion.

factors influencing protein metabolism. If the amino acid profile in the feed closely matches the horse's requirements for individual amino acids, the horse can better utilize the protein. Protein from forages is relatively poorly digested in the small intestine, whereas protein from concentrate feed is more thoroughly digested. Since a significant portion of the protein in forages is bound within the plant's structural components, it needs to be released through microbial fermentation in the hindgut. When protein is introduced into the horse's hindgut, it becomes a valuable resource for the resident gut microbes. These microorganisms possess the capability to break down and digest the protein, effectively using it as a source of energy and nutrients to fuel their own growth and metabolic processes. This microbial activity in the hindgut is a natural and essential aspect of the horse's digestive process.

Excessive protein intake in a horse's diet can result in an increase in the excretion of urea in their urine. Urea is a nitrogen-containing waste product produced because of protein metabolism in the body. When the horse consumes more protein than it can efficiently utilize, the excess nitrogen is converted into urea and excreted in the urine. This can serve as an indicator of protein overconsumption and the potential for elevated nitrogen waste levels in the horse's system. Additionally, as some specific amino acids stimulate insulin secretion, a study found a very high-protein meal led to elevated plasma insulin levels in healthy horses. The intake of a high-protein meal may impact plasma amino acid levels and trigger excessive insulin release, which could be important for horses with equine metabolic syndrome (Loos et al., 2019).

Fat digestion in the small intestine

Fat digestion in horses primarily takes place in the small intestine, specifically in the duodenum and jejunum. When a horse consumes fats, they undergo emulsification in the stomach, breaking down into smaller droplets. In the duodenum, bile salts further break down these droplets into micelles, enhancing accessibility for enzymatic digestion. Pancreatic lipase, an enzyme produced by the pancreas, then acts on these micelles, converting them into absorbable fatty acids and glycerol (Figure 1.7) (Cunha, 1991). These smaller molecules are absorbed through the intestinal walls into the bloodstream, providing the horse with a valuable source of energy and nutrients for various bodily functions.

Bile is continuously produced, and the excretion of bile salts relies on an intact enterohepatic circulation, which is necessary for fat digestion. Our understanding of fat assimilation is limited, but equine pancreatic tissue contains relatively high levels of lipase (Lorenzo-Figueras et al., 2007). Consequently, the breakdown of fat results in the formation of 2-monoacylglycerides and long-chain fatty acids. Bile salts are essential for the transportation of these products into enterocytes (Lengsfeld et al., 2004). Studies have shown that a high-fat diet (8%) does not affect pancreatic lipase activity, and even concentrations as high as 15% in adapted horses have no impact on fat digestion in the small intestine (Landes & Meyer, 1998).

It is essential to maintain a balanced fat intake in the horse's diet to support their overall health and performance. Any potential interactions between added dietary fat and nutrient digestibility could impact the determination of digestible energy and nutrient values in horse diets. The inclusion of fat in horse diets might reduce behavior issues and enhance athletic performance (Holland et al., 1998) and has been shown to reduce the risk of tying up (McKenzie, 2003). When introducing a higher-fat diet to horses, there is typically an adaptation period required to allow their digestive system and metabolism to adjust to the increased fat intake. This adaptation period can vary from horse to horse but generally spans 14 to 28 days (Julen et al., 1995).

1.2 Hindgut anatomy and digestion

The hindgut, which includes the cecum, large colon, small colon, and rectum, is rich in microorganisms. The composition of the microbiota in the hindgut, including protozoa, fungi, and bacteria, reflects the health of the gastrointestinal tract and its specific location within the hindgut (Al Jassim & Andrews, 2009). While mucus is secreted by glands in the large intestine, there are no digestive enzymes present (Frape, 2010). Interestingly, despite variations in the upper gastrointestinal tract, the populations of microorganisms in the lumen and mucosa of the lower gastrointestinal tract are remarkably consistent.

The composition of the diet and feeding practices significantly affect the microbiota and its functioning in the large intestine (Merritt & Julliand, 2013; Dougal et al., 2014; Raspa et al., 2022), which has significant implications for horse feeding strategies (Figure 1.8) (Harris & Dunnett, 2018).

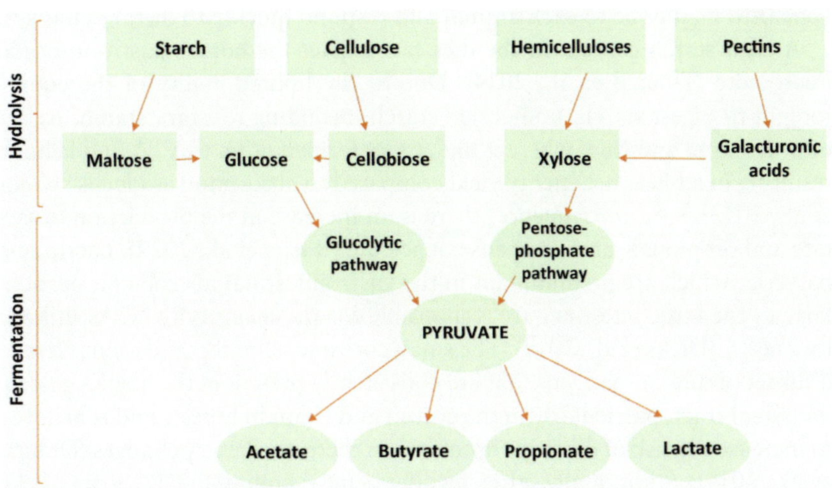

Figure 1.8 Pathways of polysaccharides hydrolysis and fermentation by the hindgut (adapted from Julliand & Grimm, 2017).

The pH in the cecum and colon is around 6.6, creating an ideal environment for anaerobic bacteria, fungi, and protozoa to break down hemicelluloses and pectins. When the pH drops below 6.0 in the large intestine, the growth of many fiber-fermenting microorganisms, such as *Ruminococcus albus* and *Fibrobacter succinogenes*, is inhibited, while acidophilic bacteria like *Streptococcus bovis*, *Lactobacillus* spp., and *Mitzuokella* spp. proliferate (Biddle et al., 2013; Milinovich et al., 2006). This leads to increased lactic acid production in the hindgut, further lowering the pH (Dicks et al., 2014), which can result in HGA, colic, and anorexia. Prolonged pH below 5.8 can cause damage to the epithelial lining and suboptimal nutrient absorption and may lead to laminitis (Dicks et al., 2014).

Efficient hindgut fermentation occurs when horses have continuous access to forage and limited exposure to feeds that may disrupt the cecal pH, such as large-grain meals or high-fructan grasses (Sadet-Bourgeteau & Julliand, 2010). In the hindgut, there is intense activity in breaking down fibrous materials, resulting in the production of VFA such as acetate, propionate, and butyrate, which serve as energy sources, and butyrate, which also supports intestinal cell health (Figure 1.9) (Varloud et al., 2004). The intensity of these fermentation processes depends on the quantity and timing of fermentable material entering from the small intestine (Merritt & Julliand, 2013). If the roughage component of the feed is kept optimal, digesta reaches the cecum and colon approximately 2–3 hours after feeding (Frape, 2010) and is fermented for 36–48 hours in the cecum (Dicks et al., 2014). The motility and capacity of the cecum increase during feeding to optimize the interaction between the bacteria and digesta (Frape, 2010). These VFAs are produced by symbiotic microbiota during the fermentation of plant-based fiber in the horse's diet. These symbiotic microbiota in the hindgut (cecum and colon) appear to be unique to each animal and respond quickly to dietary changes.

A high starch content in the diet can impact the horse's gastrointestinal microbiota (Dougal et al., 2014). Due to the limited ability of the equine foregut to digest starch, undigested starch, including resistant starch, passes into the large intestine, where it undergoes fermentation to VFA and lactate, resulting in a lower net energy yield compared to absorption as glucose (Geor et al., 2013). As a consequence, there is an increase in the production of lactate and propionate at the expense of acetate (Raspa et al., 2022). Lactic acid bacteria, which are predominant in the gastrointestinal microbiota, particularly in the large intestine, are responsible for the majority of VFAs utilized for energy (Dicks et al., 2014). The small core microfloral population refers to a subset of microorganisms that are consistently present in the horse's gastrointestinal tract, particularly in the cecum and colon in horses, and is believed to increase the risk of digestive upsets when there are dietary changes (Dougal et al., 2014). Additionally, after feeding a meal containing 1.5 g starch/kg body weight, the cecal microbiota parameters indicate that Firmicutes were the most abundant phylum, followed by Bacteroidetes, with a lower relative

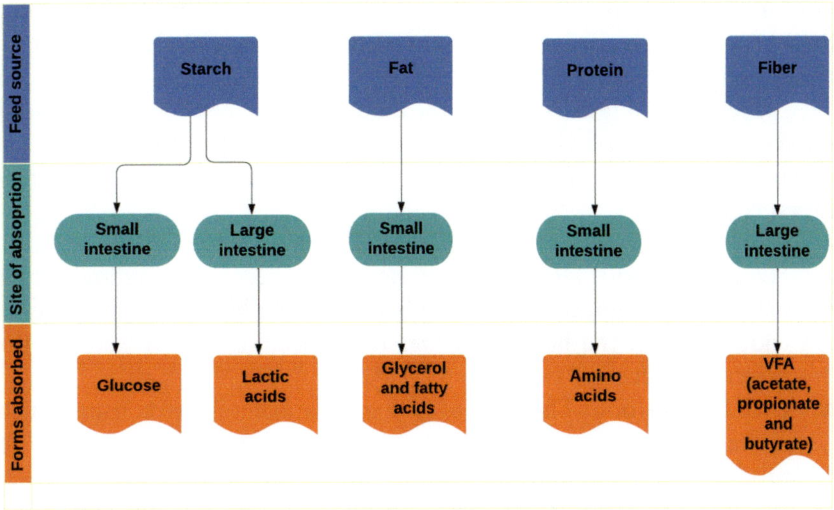

Figure 1.9 Feed sources, absorption sites, and forms in the digestive tract of horses.

abundance of Prevotella, Treponema, and Phascolarctobacterium compared to horses fed a meal with 0 g starch/kg body weight (Halpin et al., 2020).

The role of hindgut protein in contributing to the horse's amino acid pool is still a topic of debate (Merritt & Julliand, 2013). However, horses can assimilate nitrogen and amino acids from the large intestine, and growth studies using high-protein forages such as grasses or alfalfa have shown similar results to horses fed using concentrate-based protein such as soybean meal (Nash et al., 2001).

The hindgut also plays a crucial role in mineral and vitamin functions, such as the absorption of phosphorus primarily in the hindgut, absorption of sodium and chloride, synthesis of water-soluble B vitamins in the large intestine through resident microflora, and vitamin-K synthesis in the healthy large intestine (Zeyner & Harris, 2013); however, bioavailability and absorption are uncertain.

Changes in the gut microbiota can indeed have a significant influence on horses beyond just their digestive health. The gut microbiota plays a role in what is known as the gut-brain axis, a complex bidirectional communication system between the gastrointestinal tract and the central nervous system. The gastrointestinal tract, in addition to its digestive functions, secretes numerous hormones and neurotransmitters. These chemical messengers can have far-reaching effects, including on the horse's behavior and overall well-being. Disruptions in the balance of these neurotransmitters and hormonal signaling pathways can potentially lead to alterations in behavior and mood (Murphy & Bloom, 2006; Clarke et al., 2014).

The final function of the large intestine is the formation of fecal balls. As feed enters the small colon, water is absorbed, and fecal balls are formed after most of the nutrients have been extracted. Once formed, these fecal balls pass through the rectum for excretion. The transit time from ingestion to defecation, generally reported to be between 36 and 72 hours, can vary depending on factors such as the amount and fiber content of the feed offered and individual variations between horses (Raspa et al., 2022).

The water content of horse manure can vary significantly based on factors such as:

- **Hydration status:** Dehydration in horses can result in drier and firmer manure, often appearing as hard balls. When a horse doesn't consume enough water, the body conserves fluids, leading to less water in the digestive tract.
- **Diet composition:** The type of feed and forage a horse consumes can influence manure consistency. Diets high in fiber, such as hay, tend to produce bulkier and firmer manure, while diets with excessive intakes of concentrates or grains in large meals can lead to softer and looser manure related to HGA.
- **Sudden diet changes:** Abrupt changes in a horse's diet can disrupt the microbial balance in the digestive system, leading to loose manure or diarrhea. Gradual dietary transitions of a minimum of 14 days are generally recommended to minimize these problems.

Monitoring the consistency and frequency of a horse's manure can provide valuable insights into their overall health. Any persistent changes, such as very firm manure, prolonged diarrhea, or the presence of blood in the manure, should be promptly addressed by a veterinarian.

References

Alexander, F. (1966). A study of parotid salivation in the horse. *The Journal of Physiology*, *184*(3), 646–656. https://doi.org/10.1113/jphysiol.1966.sp007937

Al Jassim, R. A. M., & Andrews, F. M. (2009). The bacterial community of the horse gastrointestinal tract and its relation to fermentative acidosis, laminitis, colic, and stomach ulcers. *Veterinary Clinics of North America: Equine Practice*, *25*(2), 199–215. https://doi.org/10.1016/j.cveq.2009.04.005

Al-Rammahi, M. A. (2020). Levels of disaccharidases in the brush border membrane of equine small intestine. *Iraqi Journal of Veterinary Sciences*, *34*(1), 197–201. https://doi.org/10.33899/ijvs.2019.125778.1152

Argenzio, R. (1993). *General functions of the gastrointestinal tract and their control and integration editor WO Reece (Ed.), Duke's physiology of domestic animals* (W. O. Reece, Ed.; 11th ed.). Wiley-Blackwell.

Argenzio, R., & Stevens, C. (1975). Cyclic changes in ionic composition of digesta in the equine intestinal tract. *American Journal of Physiology-Legacy Content*, *228*(4), 1224–1230. https://doi.org/10.1152/ajplegacy.1975.228.4.1224

Baker, S. J., & Gerring, E. L. (1993). Technique for prolonged, minimally invasive monitoring of intragastric pH in ponies. *American Journal of Veterinary Research*, *54*(10), 1725–1734.

Bell, R., Mogg, T., & Kingston, J. (2007). Equine gastric ulcer syndrome in adult horses: A review. *New Zealand Veterinary Journal*, *55*(1), 1–12. https://doi.org/10.1080/00480169.2007.36728

Biddle, A. S., Black, S. J., & Blanchard, J. L. (2013). An in vitro model of the horse gut microbiome enables identification of lactate-utilizing bacteria that differentially respond to starch induction. *PLoS ONE*, *8*(10), e77599. https://doi.org/10.1371/journal.pone.0077599

Bishop, R. (2005). *The horse nutrition Bible: The comprehensive guide to the correct feeding of your horse*. David & Charles.

Bochnia, M., Boesel, M., Bahrenthien, L., Wensch-Dorendorf, M., & Zeyner, A. (2017). Feed intake patterns of sport ponies and warmblood horses following iso-energetic intake of pelleted fibre-rich mixed feed, muesli feed and semicrushed oat grains. *Journal of Animal Physiology and Animal Nutrition*, *101*(S1), 37–42. https://doi.org/10.1111/jpn.12732

Bonin, S. J., Clayton, H. M., Lanovaz, J. L., & Johnston, T. (2007). Comparison of mandibular motion in horses chewing hay and pellets. *Equine Veterinary Journal*, *39*(3), 258–262. https://doi.org/10.2746/042516407X157792

Clarke, G., Stilling, R. M., Kennedy, P. J., Stanton, C., Cryan, J. F., & Dinan, T. G. (2014). Minireview: Gut microbiota: The neglected endocrine organ. *Molecular Endocrinology*, *28*(8), 1221–1238. https://doi.org/10.1210/me.2014-1108

Colombino, E., Raspa, F., Perotti, M., Bergero, D., Vervuert, I., Valle, E., & Capucchio, M. T. (2022). Gut health of horses: Effects of high fibre vs high starch diet on histological and morphometrical parameters. *BMC Veterinary Research*, *18*(1), 338. https://doi.org/10.1186/s12917-022-03433-y

Colville, T., & Bassert, J. M. (2008). *Clinical anatomy and physiology for veterinary technicians* (2nd ed.). Mosby Elsevier.

Contreras-Aguilar, M. D., Escribano, D., Martínez-Subiela, S., Martín-Cuervo, M., Lamy, E., Tecles, F., & Cerón, J. J. (2019). Changes in saliva analytes in equine acute abdominal disease: A sialochemistry approach. *BMC Veterinary Research*, *15*(1), 187. https://doi.org/10.1186/s12917-019-1933-6

Cunha, T. J. (1991). *Horse feeding and nutrition* (2nd ed.). Academic Press.

Daly, K., Proudman, C. J., Duncan, S. H., Flint, H. J., Dyer, J., & Shirazi-Beechey, S. P. (2012). Alterations in microbiota and fermentation products in equine large intestine in response to dietary variation and intestinal disease. *British Journal of Nutrition*, *107*(7), 989–995. https://doi.org/10.1017/S0007114511003825

De Fombelle, A., Veiga, L., Drogoul, C., & Julliand, V. (2004). Effect of diet composition and feeding pattern on the prececal digestibility of starches from diverse botanical origins measured with the mobile nylon bag technique in horses. *Journal of Animal Science*, *82*(12), 3625–3634. https://doi.org/10.2527/2004.82123625x

Dicks, L. M. T., Botha, M., Dicks, E., & Botes, M. (2014). The equine gastro-intestinal tract: An overview of the microbiota, disease and treatment. *Livestock Science*, *160*, 69–81. https://doi.org/10.1016/j.livsci.2013.11.025

Dougal, K., de la Fuente, G., Harris, P. A., Girdwood, S. E., Pinloche, E., Geor, R. J., Nielsen, B. D., Schott, H. C., Elzinga, S., & Newbold, C. J. (2014). Characterisation of the faecal bacterial community in adult and elderly horses fed a high fibre, high oil or high starch diet using 454 pyrosequencing. *PLoS ONE*, *9*(2), e87424. https://doi.org/10.1371/journal.pone.0087424

Dyer, J., Merediz, E. F., Salmon, K. S. H., Proundman, C. J., Edwards, G. B., & Shirazi-Beechey, S. P. (2002). Molecular characterisation of carbohydrate digestion and absorption in equine small intestine. *Equine Veterinary Journal*, *34*(4), 349–358. https://doi.org/10.2746/042516402776249209

Ellis, A. D., Redgate, S., Zinchenko, S., Owen, H., Barfoot, C., & Harris, P. (2015). The effect of presenting forage in multi-layered haynets and at multiple sites on night time budgets of stabled horses. *Applied Animal Behaviour Science*, *171*, 108–116. https://doi.org/10.1016/j.applanim.2015.08.012

Ericsson, A. C., Johnson, P. J., Lopes, M. A., Perry, S. C., & Lanter, H. R. (2016). A microbiological map of the healthy equine gastrointestinal tract. *PLOS ONE*, *11*(11), e0166523. https://doi.org/10.1371/journal.pone.0166523

Flemström, G., & Isenberg, J. I. (2001). Gastroduodenal mucosal alkaline secretion and mucosal protection. *News in Physiological Sciences*, 16, 23–28.

Frape, D. (2004). *Equine nutrition and feeding* (3rd ed.). Wiley. https://doi.org/10.1002/9780470751053

Frape, D. (2010). *Equine nutrition and feeding* (4th ed.). Wiley-Blackwell. https://doi.org/10.1002/9780470751053

Geor, R., Harris, P., & Coenen, M. (2013). *Equine applied and clinical nutrition.* Elsevier Saunders.

Glatter, M., Borewicz, K., van den Bogert, B., Wensch-Dorendorf, M., Bochnia, M., Greef, J. M., Bachmann, M., Smidt, H., Breves, G., & Zeyner, A. (2019). Modification of the equine gastrointestinal microbiota by Jerusalem artichoke meal supplementation. *PLOS ONE*, *14*(8), e0220553. https://doi.org/10.1371/journal.pone.0220553

Greet, T. R. C. (2020). Functional anatomy and physiology of the gastrointestinal tract. *The Annual Seminar of the Equine Branch of the New Zealand Veterinary Association.*

Halpin, M. Y., Drouillard, J., Douthit, T., Ran, Q., Bradford, B. J., Marthaler, D., Ochonski, P., & Lattimer, J. M. (2020). The effect of increasing levels of dietary starch on equine cecal microbiota. *Journal of Animal Science*, *98*(Supplement 3), 21–21. https://doi.org/10.1093/jas/skaa054.036

Harris, P., & Dunnett, C. (2018). Nutritional tips for veterinarians. *Equine Veterinary Education*, *30*(9), 486–496. https://doi.org/10.1111/eve.12657

Hewetson, M., & Tallon, R. (2021). Equine squamous gastric disease: Prevalence, impact and management. *Veterinary Medicine: Research and Reports*, *12*, 381–399. https://doi.org/10.2147/VMRR.S235258

Holland, J. L., Kronfeld, D. S., Rich, G. A., Kline, K. A., Fontenot, J. P., Meacham, T. N., & Harris, P. A. (1998). Acceptance of fat and lecithin containing diets by horses. *Applied Animal Behaviour Science*, *56*(2–4), 91–96. https://doi.org/10.1016/S0168-1591(97)00101-9

Holzer, P. (1998). Neural emergency system in the stomach. *Gastroenterology*, *114*(4), 823–839. https://doi.org/10.1016/S0016-5085(98)70597-9

Husted, L., Sanchez, L. C., Olsen, S. N., Baptiste, K. E., & Merritt, A. M. (2008). Effect of paddock vs. stall housing on 24 hour gastric pH within the proximal and ventral equine stomach. *Equine Veterinary Journal*, *40*(4), 337–341. https://doi.org/10.2746/042516408X284673

Johnson, L. R. (2001). Digestion and absorption. In L. R. Johnson (Ed.), *Gastrointestinal physiology* (6th ed., pp. 119–141). CV Mosby.

Julen, T. R., Potter, G. D., Greene, L. W., & Stott, G. G. (1995). Adaptation to a fat-supplemented diet by cutting horses. *Journal of Equine Veterinary Science, 15*(10), 436–440. https://doi.org/10.1016/S0737-0806(06)81835-6

Julliand, V., De Fombelle, A., & Varloud, M. (2006). Starch digestion in horses: The impact of feed processing. *Livestock Science, 100*(1), 44–52. https://doi.org/10.1016/j.livprodsci.2005.11.001

Julliand, V., & Grimm, P. (2017). The impact of diet on the hindgut microbiome. *Journal of Equine Veterinary Science, 52*, 23–28. https://doi.org/10.1016/j.jevs.2017.03.002

Kern, D. L., Slyter, L. L., Leffel, E. C., Weaver, J. M., & Oltjen, R. R. (1974). Ponies vs. steers: Microbial and chemical characteristics of intestinal ingesta. *Journal of Animal Science, 38*(3), 559–564. https://doi.org/10.2527/jas1974.383559x

Kienzle, E., & Radicke, S. (1993). Effect of diet on maltase, sucrase and lactase in the small intestinal mucosa of the horse. *Journal of Animal Physiology and Animal Nutrition, 70*(1–5), 97–103. https://doi.org/10.1111/j.1439-0396.1993.tb00311.x

Kienzle, E., Radicke, S., Landes, E., Kleffken, D., Illenseer, M., & Meyer, H. (1994). Activity of amylase in the gastrointestinal tract of the horse. *Journal of Animal Physiology and Animal Nutrition, 72*(1–5), 234–241. https://doi.org/10.1111/j.1439-0396.1994.tb00392.x

Kitchen, D. L., Burrow, J. A., Heartless, C. S., & Merritt, A. M. (2000). Effect of pyloric blockade and infusion of histamine or pentagastrin on gastric secretion in horses. *American Journal of Veterinary Research, 61*(9), 1133–1139. https://doi.org/10.2460/ajvr.2000.61.1133

Landes, E., & Meyer, H. (1998). Influence of fat on feed intake and microbial activity in the stomach and small intestine in the horse. *Pferdeheilkunde Equine Medicine, 14*(1), 51–58. https://doi.org/10.21836/PEM19980107

Laurence, C., & Peter, R. K. (2016). *Sugars, fatty acids, and energy biochemistry.* Blackwell.

Lengsfeld, H., Beaumier-Gallon, G., Chahinian, H., De Caro, A., Verger, R., Laugier, R., & Carrière, F. (2004). Physiology of gastrointestinal lipolysis and therapeutical use of lipases and digestive lipase inhibitors. In *Lipases and phospholipases in drug development* (pp. 195–229). Wiley. https://doi.org/10.1002/3527601910.ch10

Lightbody, K. L., Matthews, J. B., Kemp-Symonds, J. G., Lambert, P. A., & Austin, C. J. (2018). Use of a saliva-based diagnostic test to identify tapeworm infection in horses in the UK. *Equine Veterinary Journal, 50*(2), 213–219. https://doi.org/10.1111/evj.12742

Lindner, A., Marx, S., Kissenbeck, S., & Mosen, H. (2000). Saliva collection and relationship between lactate concentration in blood and saliva of exercising horses. *Journal of Equine Veterinary Science, 20*(1), 52–54. https://doi.org/10.1016/S0737-0806(00)80322-6

Loos, C. M. M., Dorsch, S. C., Elzinga, S. E., Brewster-Barnes, T., Vanzant, E. S., Adams, A. A., & Urschel, K. L. (2019). A high protein meal affects plasma insulin concentrations and amino acid metabolism in horses with equine metabolic syndrome. *The Veterinary Journal*, *251*, 105341. https://doi.org/10.1016/j.tvjl.2019.105341

Lorenzo-Figueras, M., Morisset, S. M., Morisset, J., Lainé, J., & Merritt, A. M. (2007). Digestive enzyme concentrations and activities in healthy pancreatic tissue of horses. *American Journal of Veterinary Research*, *68*(10), 1070–1072. https://doi.org/10.2460/ajvr.68.10.1070

Lorenzo-Figueras, M., Preston, T., Ott, E. A., & Merritt, A. M. (2005). Meal-induced gastric relaxation and emptying in horses after ingestion of high-fat versus high-carbohydrate diets. *American Journal of Veterinary Research*, *66*(5), 897–906. https://doi.org/10.2460/ajvr.2005.66.897

Lundström, T., Lingström, P., Wattle, O., Carlén, A., & Birkhed, D. (2020). Equine saliva components during mastication, and in vivo pH changes in the oral biofilm of sound and carious tooth surfaces after sucrose exposure. *Acta Veterinaria Scandinavica*, *62*(1), 21. https://doi.org/10.1186/s13028-020-00518-2

Luthersson, N., Nielsen, K. H., Harris, P., & Parkin, T. D. H. (2009). Risk factors associated with equine gastric ulceration syndrome (EGUS) in 201 horses in Denmark. *Equine Veterinary Journal*, *41*(7), 625–630. https://doi.org/10.2746/042516409X441929

Mackie, R. I., & Wilkins, C. A. (1988). Enumeration of anaerobic bacterial microflora of the equine gastrointestinal tract. *Applied and Environmental Microbiology*, *54*(9), 2155–2160. https://doi.org/10.1128/aem.54.9.2155-2160.1988

Maisonpierre, I. N., Sutton, M. A., Harris, P., Menzies-Gow, N., Weller, R., & Pfau, T. (2019). Accelerometer activity tracking in horses and the effect of pasture management on time budget. *Equine Veterinary Journal*, *51*(6), 840–845. https://doi.org/10.1111/evj.13130

Martinson, K., Jung, H., Hathaway, M., & Sheaffer, C. (2012). The effect of soaking on carbohydrate removal and dry matter loss in orchardgrass and Alfalfa Hays. *Journal of Equine Veterinary Science*, *32*(6), 332–338. https://doi.org/10.1016/j.jevs.2011.11.009

McKenzie, E. (2003). Nutritional management of exertional Rhabdomyolysis. In *Current therapy in equine medicine* (pp. 727–734). Elsevier. https://doi.org/10.1016/B978-0-7216-9540-2.50197-3

Merritt, A. (2003). The equine stomach: A personal perspective (1963–2003). *Proc. Am. Ass. Equine Pract.*, *49*.

Merritt, A. M., & Julliand, V. (2013). Gastrointestinal physiology. In R. J. Geor, P. A. Harris, & M. Coenen (Eds.), *Equine applied and clinical nutrition* (pp. 3–32). Elsevier. https://doi.org/10.1016/B978-0-7020-3422-0.00001-8

Metayer, N., Lhote, M., Bahr, A., Cohen, N. D., Kim, I., Roussel, A. J., & Julliand, V. (2004). Meal size and starch content affect gastric emptying in horses. *Equine Veterinary Journal*, *36*(5), 436–440. https://doi.org/10.2746/0425164044868468

Meyer, H. (1985). Investigations on saliva production and chewing effects in horses fed various feeds. *Proceedings of the 9th Equine Nutrition and Physiology Symposium; 23–25 May, 1985, Michigan State University, East Lansing, MI, USA*. https://cir.nii.ac.jp/crid/1573105975030947328.bib?lang=en

Meyer, H., Ahiswedeu, L., & Reinhardt, H. J. (1975). Studies on the duration of feeding, masticatory frequency and mincing of feed in horses. *DTW. Deutsche Tierarztliche Wochenschrift*, *82*(2), 54–58.

Meyer, H., Coenen, M., & Prost, D. (1986). Digestive physiology of the horse. 14 Feed insalivation and passage in the equine upper intestinal tract. *Journal of Animal Physiology and Animal Nutrition*, *56*, 171–183.

Milinovich, G. J., Trott, D. J., Burrell, P. C., Van Eps, A. W., Thoefner, M. B., Blackall, L. L., Al Jassim, R. A. M., Morton, J. M., & Pollitt, C. C. (2006). Changes in equine hindgut bacterial populations during oligofructose-induced laminitis. *Environmental Microbiology*, *8*(5), 885–898. https://doi.org/10.1111/j.1462-2920.2005.00975.x

Moeller, B. A., McCall, C. A., Silverman, S. J., & McElhenney, W. H. (2008). Estimation of saliva production in crib-biting and normal horses. *Journal of Equine Veterinary Science*, *28*(2), 85–90. https://doi.org/10.1016/j.jevs.2008.01.006

Moran, A. W., Al-Rammahi, M. A., Batchelor, D. J., Bravo, D. M., & Shirazi-Beechey, S. P. (2018). Glucagon-like peptide-2 and the enteric nervous system are components of cell-cell communication pathway regulating intestinal Na+/Glucose co-transport. *Frontiers in Nutrition*, *5*. https://doi.org/10.3389/fnut.2018.00101

Muñoz-Prieto, A., Contreras-Aguilar, M. D., Cerón, J. J., Ayala de la Peña, I., Martín-Cuervo, M., Eckersall, P. D., Holm Henriksen, I.-M., Tecles, F., & Hansen, S. (2023). Changes in calprotectin (S100A8-A9) and aldolase in the saliva of horses with equine gastric ulcer syndrome. *Animals*, *13*(8), 1367. https://doi.org/10.3390/ani13081367

Murphy, K. G., & Bloom, S. R. (2006). Gut hormones and the regulation of energy homeostasis. *Nature*, *444*(7121), 854–859. https://doi.org/10.1038/nature05484

Murray, M. J., & Mahaffey, E. A. (1993). Age-related characteristics of gastric squamous epithelial mucosa in foals. *Equine Veterinary Journal*, *25*(6), 514–517. https://doi.org/10.1111/j.2042-3306.1993.tb03003.x

Nash, D. G., Avery, A., Dempsey, W., & Nash, G. (2001). Growth and development of young Thoroughbred horses on temperate Australian pastures. *Proceedings of the 17th Equine Nutrition and Physiology Symposium*, 196–198.

Nickel, R., Schummer, A., Seiferle, E., & Sack, W. O. (1979). *The viscera of the domestic mammals*. Springer. https://doi.org/10.1007/978-1-4757-6814-5

Pagan, J. D. (1998). *Advances in equine nutrition* (1st ed.). Nottingham University Press, 50–51.

Perkins, G. A., den Bakker, H. C., Burton, A. J., Erb, H. N., McDonough, S. P., McDonough, P. L., Parker, J., Rosenthal, R. L., Wiedmann, M., Dowd, S. E., & Simpson, K. W. (2012). Equine stomachs harbor an abundant and diverse mucosal microbiota. *Applied and Environmental Microbiology*, *78*(8), 2522–2532. https://doi.org/10.1128/AEM.06252-11

Pfeiffer, C. J., & Dabareiner, R. M. (1992). Ultrastructure of Brunner's glands in the horse. *Journal of Submicroscopic Cytology and Pathology*, *24*(4), 581–588.

Potter, G., Arnold, F., Householder, D., Hansen, D., & Bowen, K. (1992). Digestion of starch in the small or large intestine of the equine. *European Conference on Horse Nutrition*, 109–111.

Raspa, F., Vervuert, I., Capucchio, M. T., Colombino, E., Bergero, D., Forte, C., Greppi, M., Cavallarin, L., Giribaldi, M., Antoniazzi, S., Cavallini, D., Valvassori, E., & Valle, E. (2022). A high-starch vs. high-fibre diet: Effects on the gut environment of the different intestinal compartments of the horse digestive tract. *BMC Veterinary Research*, *18*(1), 187. https://doi.org/10.1186/s12917-022-03289-2

Richards, N., Choct, M., Hinch, G. N., & Rowe, J. B. (2004). Examination of the use of exogenous α-amylase and amyloglucosidase to enhance starch digestion in the small intestine of the horse. *Animal Feed Science and Technology*, *114*(1–4), 295–305. https://doi.org/10.1016/j.anifeedsci.2003.09.004

Roberts, M. C. (1975). Carbohydrate digestion and absorption in the equine small intestine. *Journal of the South African Veterinary Association*, *46*(1), 19–27.

Röder, P. V., Geillinger, K. E., Zietek, T. S., Thorens, B., Koepsell, H., & Daniel, H. (2014). The role of SGLT1 and GLUT2 in intestinal glucose transport and sensing. *PLoS ONE*, *9*(2), e89977. https://doi.org/10.1371/journal.pone.0089977

Sadet-Bourgeteau, S., & Julliand, V. (2010). Equine microbial gastro-intestinal health. *EAAP Scientific Series*, *128*, 161–182.

Sandberg, D. C., & Flythe, M. D. (2016). The effects of fiber sources on equine cecal fermentation. *Journal of Animal Science*, *94*(3), 1100–1107.

Van Weyenberg, S., Sales, J., & Janssens, G. P. J. (2006). Passage rate of digesta through the equine gastrointestinal tract: A review. *Livestock Science*, *99*(1), 3–12. https://doi.org/10.1016/j.livprodsci.2005.04.008

Varloud, M. (2006). *Activité amylolytique des secretions salivaires. In: Implication des microorganismes de l'estomac dans la digestion de l'amidon par le cheval.* National Agricultural Institute of Paris-Grignon.

Varloud, M., Fombelle, A. de, Goachet, A. G., Drogoul, C., & Julliand, V. (2004). Partial and total apparent digestibility of dietary carbohydrates in horses as affected by the diet. *Animal Science*, *79*(1), 61–72. https://doi.org/10.1017/S1357729800054539

Varloud, M., Roussel, A., Boisot, P., & Julliand, V. (2007). A technique for the collection and the study of biochemical and microbial characteristics of postprandial gastric contents from conscious horses. *Animal Feed Science and Technology*, *133*(3–4), 259–274. https://doi.org/10.1016/j.anifeedsci.2006.04.004

Wise, J. C., Raidal, S. L., Wilkes, E. J. A., & Hughes, K. J. (2020). Intragastric pH of foals admitted to the intensive care unit. *Journal of Veterinary Internal Medicine*, *34*(6), 2719–2726. https://doi.org/10.1111/jvim.15888

Zeyner, A., & Harris, P. A. (2013). Vitamins. In R. J. Geor, P. A. Harris, & M. Coenen (Eds.), *Equine clinical and applied nutrition* (pp. 168–189). Elsevier.

CHAPTER 2

Feed sources for horses

Feeding a horse is an individual process because nutrient requirements differ from individual to individual and are influenced by the horse's breed, age, body mass, workload, and metabolic efficiency. When feeding horses, it is essential to remember that the recommended daily allowances of six basic nutrient categories must be met: carbohydrates, protein, fat, vitamins, minerals, and water. Most horses require a very simple diet to meet their nutritional needs.

Forage and concentrates are the main types of feedstuffs used in horse diets. Forage plants include plants that can be grazed or processed, such as pasture, hay, haylage, super fibers, and straw. Concentrates can contain cereal grains such as maize, barley, oats, grain by-products, and protein sources, plus some forage. In addition, additivities such as protein supplements, vitamin and mineral mixes, probiotics, prebiotics, joint supplements, and herbs are currently available on the market and widely used in horse diets. The most common feed sources will be explained in this section so that they can be used optimally in creating rations.

2.1 Forage

The horse is a grazing animal, designed to eat almost constantly throughout the day. Horses are herbivorous, and their digestive system is designed to suit a grazing lifestyle and eat almost constantly throughout the day. Their natural diet consists of grasses and plants, and they have evolved to eat for up to 18 hours per day. Forage is defined as a fiber-rich feedstuff (structural carbohydrate), and the recent advances in equine nutrition

DOI: 10.1201/9781003379355-2

research recommend more plant-fiber and forage-based diets for horses (Harris et al., 2017).

The advantages of feeding forage to horses

- Forage is a source of fiber which is required to keep a horse's digestive system functioning properly.
- It is a source of slow-release energy from slow fermentation in the hindgut. The microbial fermentation of fiber in the hindgut is a slow and steady process. This gradual fermentation of forage fiber results in volatile fatty acids (VFAs) as a by-product. These VFAs provide a consistent source of energy to the horse, even when the horse is not eating.
- It supports healthy hindgut microflora. The horse has a well-developed symbiotic relationship with the hindgut microbiota, which ferments the forage fibers (Muhonen et al., 2021).
- Forage increases the chewing rate, and therefore reduces the risk of stereotypic behaviors, particularly crib biting or wood chewing.
- Feeding forage to horses reduces the risk of equine gastric ulcer syndrome, as they spend more time chewing and produce large amounts of saliva, which helps to buffer the acid that is produced in the stomach.
- Forage reduces the risk of hindgut disturbances and acidosis (HGA). The slow, fiber-based fermentation of forage minimizes the production of lactic acid, which is a key contributor to hindgut acidosis.
- It reduces the risk of behavior abnormalities due to its relatively low levels of non-structural carbohydrates, as these can lead to hindgut disturbances.

Understanding forage digestion in comparison to grain digestion in horses

The majority of fibrous feeds are digested in the hindgut. Microbial fermentation in the hindgut produces VFAs, which are organic compounds such as acetic acid, propionic acid, and butyric acid. VFAs are primarily associated with fiber fermentation in the horse's hindgut, particularly the cecum and colon. These energy-producing substrates are easily absorbed into the bloodstream, and they are converted to glucose, fat, or used directly as an energy source. Diet has a significant impact on the concentrations of acetate, propionate, and butyrate, and the number and type of microorganisms in the hindgut. It is critical to provide enough fiber to keep those microorganisms healthy.

Grain feeding should be kept to a minimum because grain is mostly made up of hydrolyzable carbohydrates (starch) and variable amounts of fiber. However, horses' digestive systems are not well adapted to digest starch, which is a complex compound composed of many bonded glucose molecules. During starch digestion, an enzyme called amylase breaks down starch primarily in the horse's small intestine.

Dietary differences in fiber and starch affect short-chain fatty acids and lactate concentrations, and the hindgut digesta's capacity to buffer lactate impacts the horse's digesta pH and hindgut health (Muhonen et al., 2021). If the horse's diet is high in starch, their small intestine cannot digest all of the starch, and undigested starch passes through to the hindgut, resulting in a lower colon and/or cecal pH level, described as hindgut acidosis. This can increase the risk of health issues such as colic or laminitis.

Factors influencing fiber intake and digestibility in horses

Multiple factors influence fiber intake and digestibility, including crude protein (CP), acid detergent fiber (ADF), neutral detergent fiber (NDF), and lignin concentrations. Higher CP concentrations have been associated with increased intake and digestibility, but have not been well documented within forage species in horses (Moore et al., 1999).

The original system of analyzing the "fibrous" fraction of feedstuffs includes measuring crude fiber. Thus, crude fiber extract was used as a reference for fibrous components, or the indigestible portion of carbohydrates in feed. Some of these components, however, are partially fermentable by microorganisms in the hindgut of horses. As a result, equine nutritionists have abandoned the crude fiber assay in favor of the detergent fiber analysis system, as follows:

- **The acid detergent fiber** indicates the amount of cellulose and lignin in a plant, and it is often used to indirectly measure forage digestibility. Cellulose can be used as an energy source by animals in part, but lignin cannot. Lignin also has a big negative impact on fiber digestibility, and as a plant matures, the ADF (cellulose and lignin) level rises, reducing digestibility.
- **The neutral detergent fiber**, a measure of total cell wall content including hemicellulose, cellulose, and lignin, increases as the plant matures, and is used to predict intake potential. Immature hay, cut earlier in the season, is easier for horses to digest because it has a lower ADF percentage, and it is also more easily consumed because it has a lower NDF percentage. Hemicellulose is more digestible than ADF components in the large intestine of the horse.

Furthermore, soluble fiber content and non-structural carbohydrates have a significant impact on fiber digestibility in horses.

- **Soluble fiber:** Some forage components, such as pectins and gums, are classified as soluble fibers. Microbes in the hindgut easily ferment these fibers, providing an additional source of energy. They do so, however, at a slower and more controlled rate than simple sugars because their fermentation promotes the production of beneficial VFAs without the rapid production of lactic acid, contributing to hindgut stability and reducing the risk of acidosis.

- **Non-structural carbohydrates (NSCs):** NSCs are the carbohydrates in the diet that are easily digestible, such as sugars and starches. Forages typically contain fewer NSCs than grains. Feeding diets high in NSCs, such as grains, can increase the risk of hindgut acidosis because these carbohydrates may not be fully digested in the small intestine and are fermented more quickly, resulting in a drop in pH level and reduced fiber-digestive efficiency.

Pasture

Pasture is the most important feed in many horses' diets. Horses' two pairs of incisors enable them to graze more selectively and closer to the ground than ruminants (Hongo & Akimoto, 2003). It has been widely demonstrated that grazing intensity impacts plant diversity; moderate grazing can induce a spatial heterogeneity favorable to plant diversity (McNaughton, 1984).

What is a latrine area?

Horses are spot grazers. They overgraze some areas of a pasture and defecate in others (Figure 2.1). If feces are not removed from the pasture regularly, horses will create latrine areas where excreta and nutrients accumulate because they actively avoid grazing where they defecate, resulting in patches of long grass and weeds. In addition, horse manure tends to accumulate phosphorus in latrine areas, a factor recognized for favoring certain plant species over others and reducing overall species diversity (Ceulemans et al., 2011). Failing to promptly remove feces from pastures may increase the risk of parasitic infections and larvae.

Horse pastures typically consist of various grasses, legumes, and other plant species. There are two kinds of forage grasses (Table 2.1):

- **Cool-season grasses** found in temperate regions begin growth when temperatures reach 7°C, with optimal growth occurring between 16°C and 24°C (Geor et al., 2013), and they are often referred to as "northern grasses" in the Northern hemisphere. Cool-season grasses undergo C3 photosynthesis. The most common are Kentucky bluegrass (*Poa*

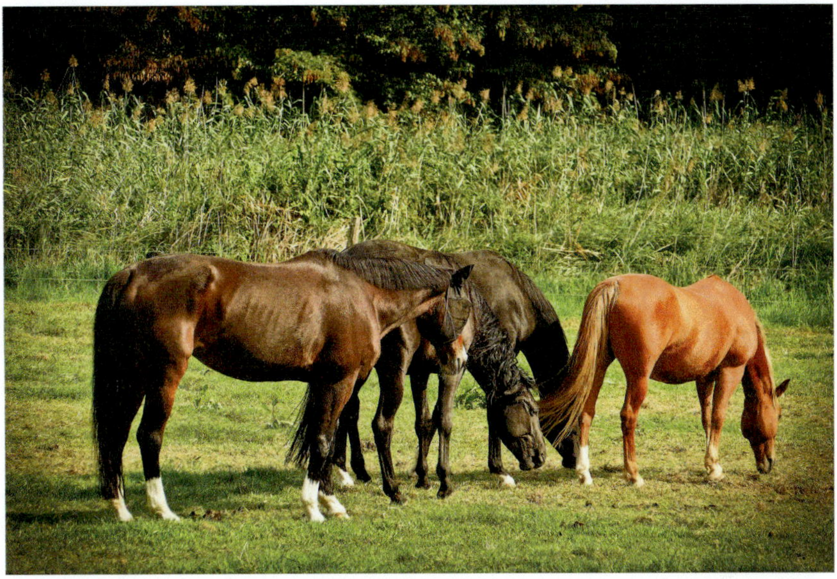

Figure 2.1 Pasture overgrazed by horses.

Table 2.1 The main differences between warm- and cool-season grasses

Factors	*Warm-season grasses*	*Cool-season grasses*
Major storage carbohydrates	Starch	Sugars including fructan
Maturity	Rapid maturity	
Cell wall content	More cell wall and lignin	
Non-structural carbohydrates	Less	More
Protein level	Less	More
Digestibility	Less	More digestible

pratensis), timothy (*Phleum pretense*), meadow fescue (*Festuca pratensis*), tall fescue (*Festuca arundinacea*), perennial ryegrass (*Lolium perenne*), and cocksfoot/orchard grass (*Dactylis glomerata*). Cool-season grasses are generally more digestible than warm-season varieties. Additionally, cool-season grasses typically contain higher levels of NSC, which includes higher fructan content.

- **Warm-season grasses** found in subtropical regions begin growth at around 15°C, with optimal growth occurring between 32°C and 35°C (Geor et al., 2013), and they are often called "southern grasses." Warm-season grasses undergo C4 photosynthesis. The most common are bermudagrass (*Cynodon dactylon*), bahiagrass (*Paspalum notatum*), and dallisgrass/paspalum (*Paspalum dilatatum*).

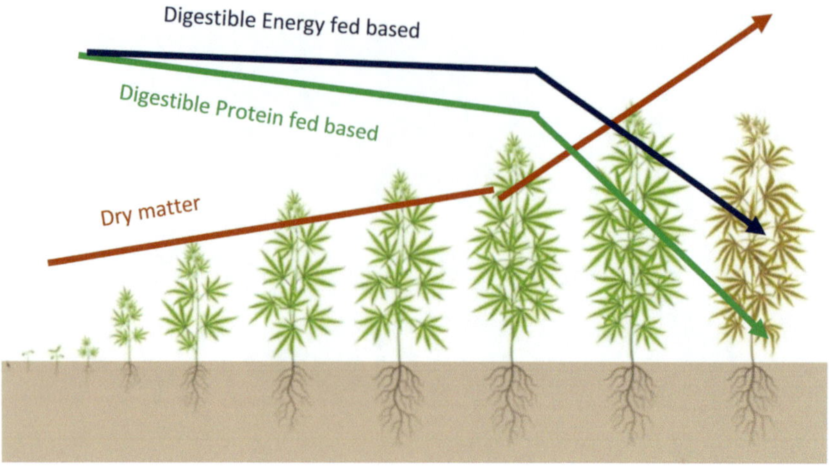

Figure 2.2 A schematic illustration of the maturation of plants and the effect on dry-matter content, digestible energy, and digestible protein content on as fed basis (Harris et al., 2017).

Warm-season grasses tend to mature faster than cool-season grasses, which can lead to reduced digestibility. Moreover, they may contain elevated levels of oxalates, which can hinder the digestibility of calcium. However, it's important to note that they generally do not contain fructans.

The horse's natural diet, grass from pasture, undergoes seasonal variation in its soluble (hydrolyzable) carbohydrate and protein content (Hoffman et al., 2001). The extent of the maturation of plants and the effect on nutrients may be affected by environmental conditions as well as management practices. Plant maturity is an important determinant of forage digestibility, with digestibility decreasing with lower protein and energy content and increasing with lower leaf-to-stem ratios during reproductive development and stem elongation (NRC, 2007) (Figure 2.2).

Factors influencing grass chemical composition

- **Plant maturity:** As grasses mature, their nutritional quality generally declines (Evans, 1995). Plants generally decrease in simple sugars and CP content and increase in fiber content as they mature. As plants produce seed heads, the starch content may increase as well (Chatterton et al., 2006).
- **Effect of season:** The circadian and seasonal variation of carbohydrates in forage is subject to "ideal" conditions and varies due to light intensity, temperature, soil, and water. For instance, orchard grass (*Dactylis glomerata*), a perennial cool-season grass frequently employed in pastures and for hay production, may respond to drought by enhancing

its sugar production (Volaire & Lelièvre, 1997). Consequently, this response can result in elevated levels of NSC within the plant.

- **Effect of time of day:** The cool-season forages utilize soluble carbohydrates produced from photosynthesis, typically resulting in the lowest NSC content in the early morning, which then peaks in the late afternoon and declines through the overnight hours as respiration utilizes the soluble carbohydrates (Williams et al., 2019).

Grazing

Due to their nutritional characteristics, horses are adapted to continuously intake small amounts of forage. Horses show numerous feeding periods (making a total of 10–18 hours) within a day. Many horses are kept in stables or yards and are unable to exhibit their natural grazing behavior; however, a sufficient daily amount of forage is essential for ensuring behavioral, physical, physiological, and mental well-being (Baumgartner et al., 2020).

There are five grazing systems commonly used with horses

- **Continuous grazing:** Continuous grazing is a simple method of allowing animals to graze in one pasture without resting periods. If animals are removed from the pasture at any given point during the season, the system is interrupted and may then be called pseudo-continuous grazing (Bott et al., 2013). Continuous grazing often results in underutilization of forage, as horses prefer to return to young, growing plants and tend to leave older plants (Henning, 2000), since the nutritive value of forage decreases as the plant matures. Continuous grazing systems have a less uniform distribution of animal defecation than those that implement rotational systems (Henning, 2000), contributing to an overload of nutrients such as phosphorus in some areas of the pasture. Horses are selective grazers and if allowed to graze forages continuously, they will repeatedly re-graze and/or overgraze plants, resulting in shorter, often defoliated swards, while leaving other ungrazed areas as "eliminative" or "latrine" areas. A recent study showed that a difference in the forage sward height of the two systems was evident, with the continuously grazed pastures having shorter sward heights than the rotationally grazed pastures (Williams et al., 2019).
- **Rotational grazing:** A rotational grazing system comprises a series of pastures that are used at various times, on a rotational basis, based on weather and forage availability. In a rotational grazing system, a group of animals is moved from one pasture to the next, to allow for rest and regrowth periods and maximize forage production (Figure 2.3). After rotation to another pasture, the previously grazed pasture is allowed to regrow to 15 to 20 cm, allowing for maintenance through mowing,

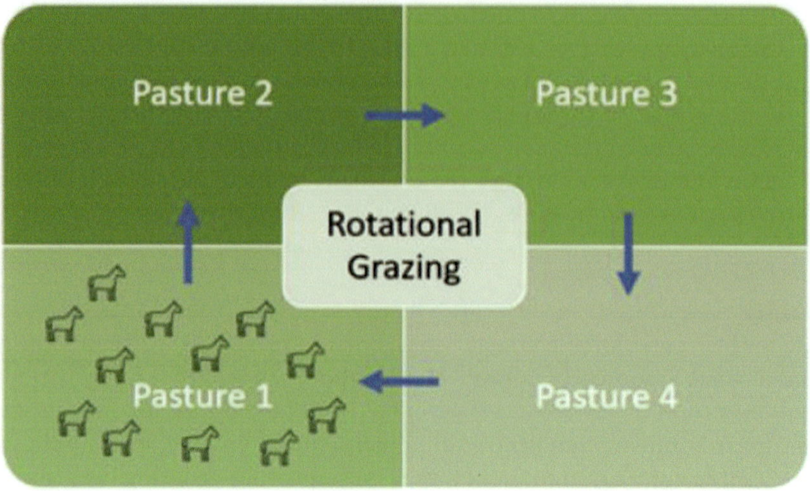

Figure 2.3 Rotational grazing on pasture.

fertilizing, and/or harrowing prior to allowing horses to return to grazing (Bott et al., 2013). Horses used in a rotational grazing scheme are not given the opportunity to be overly selective, thus grazing forages uniformly and closely before being transferred to another pasture, thereby allowing for optimal use of the pasture. Horses allowed to graze continuously tend to re-graze short, immature plants while leaving plants in eliminative areas to mature. Proper rotational grazing should leave enough ungrazed forage to allow for quick recovery and high productivity. In rotational grazing systems, forage should be rested and allowed to grow to the recommended height of 15–20 cm or higher (Henning et al., 2000; Undersander et al., 2002) before grazing again. Rotational grazing by horses is associated with better forage quality and greater pasture productivity, evidenced by higher concentrations of digestible energy (DE) and NSC, and lower levels of fiber fractions (ADF, NDF, and lignin) compared to continuous grazing (Daniel et al., 2015).

- **Strip grazing:** Horse owners have used strip grazing in various forms for decades, but there has been little work looking at how effective such a practice is. Strip grazing involves fencing off a small area (or strip) in your horse's field and moving it regularly to allow access to fresh grass. The easiest way to set it up is with temporary electric fencing – how often you move this fencing will depend on the grass growth and how much your horse needs to consume, which will vary throughout the year. When the grass has been eaten down, move the fence lines by approximately 1 m. This will open part of the resting section to become part of the grazing area, while allowing another part to become part of the recovery section. Restricting grass intake is an essential part of many weight-management programs, but is strip grazing an effective solution? Recent research showed that under controlled conditions, strip grazing can reduce the rate of weight gain in ponies living out at pasture; therefore, it can be used in weight-management programs as an effective solution to limit pasture intake (Longland, Barfoot, et al., 2011).

- **Multispecies grazing:** In order to more efficiently utilize pastures, multispecies grazing may be used. Grazing cattle in the same pasture as horses, or shortly after horses have been removed from a pasture, has been reported to be an effective use of the pasture for horse owners who also raise cattle (Bott et al., 2013). Another study (Schmitz et al., 2020) monitored grassland vegetation in West Central Germany and compared paddocks grazed by horses under two different regimes, continuous and rotational, to paddocks grazed by cattle under similar trophic site conditions. There were more plant species and more high-nature-value indicator species on continuous-grazing paddocks compared to paddocks grazed by cattle. The vegetation of paddocks grazed by cattle was more tolerant to grazing and had higher forage value than continuous grazing. This study demonstrated the potential of horse grazing to maintain species richness of temperate grasslands, as it did not confirm increasing risks of the nature value of the horse-grazed grasslands. In particular, continuous grazing with horses led to a pronounced floristic contrast within paddocks, and species richness at the paddock scale was strongly related to this plant diversity.
- **Part-time grazing:** Horses are less adapted to short access time to pasture, but this is a common practice with many horses and ponies. Part-time grazing (PTG) is the grazing technique based on the time-restricted access to pasture of farmed herbivores, usually supplemented indoors (Molle et al., 2022). Nevertheless, due to lower-fiber chewing, fiber digestibility could be reduced, particularly with limited access time where rapid pasture intake has been demonstrated. Ponies prone to obesity and laminitis have been shown to eat more than half their daily drymatter (DM) requirements in just a few hours (Longland et al., 2011). In general, PTG can improve horse health and welfare as compared with stall-feeding with reference to appropriate behavior and freedom from risks of stable vices and other pathologies.

Grazing horses have the potential to negatively affect the soil and herbage characteristics of an area, including weeds, water sources, and invertebrate populations (Bott et al., 2013). It has been widely demonstrated that grazing intensity impacts plant diversity; moderate grazing can induce a spatial heterogeneity favorable to plant diversity (McNaughton, 1984).

In temperate grasslands, the grazing regime, i.e., continuous or rotational grazing, can modify the grazer's effect on the pasture vegetation. Under continuous grazing, grazers have unrestricted access to a paddock during prolonged periods of the grazing season, which promotes the development of distinct patches of short and tall grass (Singer et al., 2001). In contrast, under rotational grazing, access to the grazing area is limited in time and space, which leads to more uniform grazing (Williams et al., 2019).

Perennial cool-season grasses store reserve soluble carbohydrates (like sugars, including fructans) in the base of the stem (White, 1973), so the repeated close grazing observed in continuously grazed pastures theoretically exposes horses to these portions high in soluble carbohydrates. However, taller swards in clipped pastures have been shown to have higher soluble carbohydrates (including starch) than short swards (Siciliano et al., 2017). White (1973) concluded that grazing can be more detrimental to pastures than mowing or mulching due to animals' selective grazing patterns.

Grazing efficiency rate

It is essential to recognize that stocking density, soil fertility, and plant species collectively determine the nutritive potential of a pasture, not just the grazing system used. Grazing selectivity is negatively correlated to stocking rate; as animals are stocked more densely, they must compete for limited forage resources and cannot afford to be as selective. If a 500-kg horse eats 3% body weight (BW) per day (15 kg per day) over 180 days, then the total forage required during that period is 270 kg, or 0.9–1.6 ha/horse. Assuming grazing efficiency rates ranging between 40% and 70%; 1724–3017 kg/ha are available for grazing. This value varies greatly depending on region, weather conditions, and agronomic management (Bott et al., 2013).

Grass consumption

There is little data on horses' voluntary dry-matter intake (VDMI) of fresh forage, due to the difficulties in measuring intakes by grazing animals. Grass intakes as high as 5.2% BW (456 g DM/kg$^{0.75}$ for a 500-kg horse) have been reported (Smith et al., 2007). Ponies grazing autumn pastures consumed 0.8% of their BW as DM in 3 hours (Longland et al., 2011). VDMI for horses varies by category, with weanlings and lactating mares eating the most. It can be concluded that the average DM intake of fresh forage is 1.8%–3% of BW, as frequently reported and thus used in practice (Edouard et al., 2008; NRC, 2007).

Grazing muzzles are essential equipment in equine management, particularly in situations where it is necessary to restrict a horse's grass intake. In a recent study specifically involving ponies, the results were remarkable, showing an average reduction of 79% in their pasture consumption

(Longland, Barfoot, et al., 2011). Such findings emphasize the vital role that grazing muzzles play in controlling and managing horses' diets, helping to prevent issues related to overconsumption of grass, obesity, and metabolic disorders. The design of the grazing muzzle and the height of the pasture sward will determine how effectively the muzzle reduces DM intake.

Hay

Grass hays, such as meadow hay, are widely used as the main forage for horses globally. However, the specific types of hay fed to horses can vary depending on the geographical area and local feeding traditions. It is important to consider the individual needs of horses when selecting the appropriate type of hay, as there is no universally best hay for all horses.

Meadow hay is derived from permanent pasture and typically consists of a mix of grasses, including clover, timothy, ryegrass, herbs, and wildflowers. It is known for its softer texture and generally higher digestibility compared to seed hay.

Legume hays, such as alfalfa/lucerne or clover, are derived from plants that can fix nitrogen from the soil, which is an important component of protein. As a result, legume hays generally have higher protein and DE content, as well as increased calcium levels, compared to most grass hays. Alfalfa is known to have a buffering effect on the acid in the stomach and hindgut.

The selection of the type of hay should be based on the specific nutritional requirements and individual needs of horses to ensure they achieve optimal health and well-being. Plant maturity affects the cell wall and cell wall contents, as well as other nutritional values (Table 2.2). Hay typically has lower nutritional value than fresh grass due to several factors.

Table 2.2 The impact of forage maturity on nutritional values

Plant maturity ↑	*Cell content* ↓	*Cell wall content* ↑
	Leaf-to-stem ratio	Water-binding capacity
	Non-structural carbohydrate level	Lignification level
	Protein and trace minerals content	Dry-matter content
	Storage carbohydrates level	Fiber content
	*Digestibility	

*Digestibility decreases as the maturity of the plant increases, is generally accurate, and applies to various types of grass hay, including timothy, rye, and bermudagrass. Early cuts are typically softer, more palatable, and have higher digestibility. As the plants mature and accumulate more fibrous material like lignin, the digestibility decreases.

- Dry hay tends to have a higher proportion of stems and fewer leaves. Leaves contain more nutrients, but they also dry out faster than stems, leading to the loss of nutritious leaf material.
- Hay has a lower NSC content, particularly water-soluble carbohydrates. After cutting, plant respiration continues, which contributes to nutrient loss, especially in terms of NSC.
- The CP content in dry hay is lower than in fresh grass. This decrease in protein content is a result of proteolysis, a process that increases the presence of non-protein nitrogen and alters the amino acid profile.
- Hay has lower levels of certain vitamins, including beta-carotene, vitamin E, and vitamin K, while the vitamin D content may be higher. It also has lower levels of omega-3 fatty acids. These losses increase as the hay ages.
- Hay typically has a higher fiber content compared to fresh grass. As forage matures, there is a decrease in the cell content and an increase in the cell wall content, leading to variations in nutritive value.
- Hay that is wet from rain after being cut will have lower nutritional values, especially NSC and energy, and be more prone to mold and mycotoxin contamination.

It is important to consider these factors and choose hay that meets the specific nutritional needs of horses, especially when fresh grass is unavailable. Regular assessment of the forage's quality and nutritional composition can help ensure that horses receive the necessary nutrients for their overall health and performance.

There are various types of hay, each with its own nutritional value and palatability. Oaten hay is known for its nutritional richness and appealing taste, and is often commended for its well-balanced combination of dietary fiber and protein. The quality and digestibility of oaten hay can be influenced by the timing of its harvest.

In practice, what role do haynets play in horse nutrition and feeding?

Providing forage in haynets has been found to prolong the time horses spend eating and slow down their rate of forage consumption compared to feeding forage directly on the floor. It can also reduce wastage but may disadvantage respiratory health in that horses are not eating hay with their head and neck down. When horses have limited access to forage, they tend to spend less time eating or foraging, which can have negative implications for their welfare. Therefore, finding strategies to maximize foraging time is important. Recent research by Lundqvist & Elisabeth Muller (2022) suggests two potential approaches:

- Using small-hole haynets can reduce the rate at which horses consume forage.

- Adding straw to the forage has been found to extend the total feeding time in horses.

By implementing these strategies, horse owners and caregivers can promote longer and more natural feeding behaviors, which may positively impact the well-being of the animals (Lundqvist & Elisabeth Müller, 2022) (Figure 2.4).

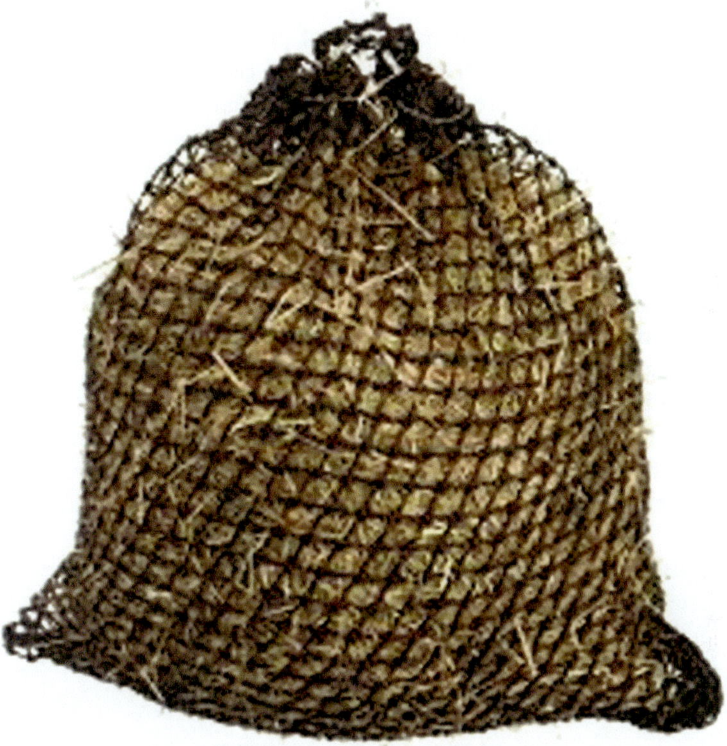

Figure 2.4 Haynet for horses.

Legume hays: Alfalfa and clover

Alfalfa is one of the most protein-rich plant-based forages. It has a high protein content, typically greater than 17%, and is high in energy. Alfalfa's flavor is highly appealing to horses, making it a popular forage source. In general, legumes have a lower fiber content than grasses, but they also contain more lignified and less digestible fiber. Legume forages, like lucerne, have a high pectin content, which is a complex carbohydrate that is rapidly degraded and not fermented into lactate (Van Soest et al., 1991). Compared to grass hays, clover hay typically has a greater protein content and is generally well-eaten by horses, although it can be more prone to mold and mycotoxin contamination. Various varieties of clover hay are available, including red clover hay and white clover hay. The inclusion of clover in a grass hay will increase protein and calcium content.

Alternative forage sources

Historically, the most common method of preserving forage was sun drying in the field to produce hay. However, the risk of poor nutritional and hygienic hay quality is present in many European countries with inclement weather during harvest and drying. This has been replaced over time by preservation by ensiling, which is based on the principle of anaerobic fermentation.

Haylage: Hay is forage preserved with a DM content greater than 85%. Haylage is a form of preserved forage that is tightly stored and has a DM content greater than 50%. The forage is chopped into smaller pieces after harvesting to make haylages. The chopped forage is tightly packed into large plastic or plastic-wrapped packages (Figure 2.5). The packing process must exclude as much oxygen as possible because oxygen can cause spoilage. When oxygen is removed from the environment, the natural fermentation process begins. Lactic acid bacteria convert forage sugars into lactic acid, lowering the pH and preserving the forage. This procedure typically

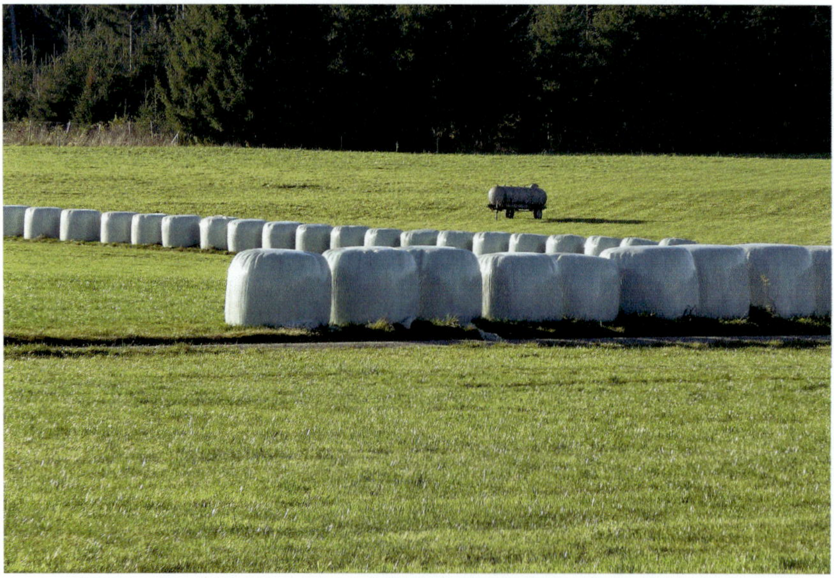

Figure 2.5 Haylage bales in plastic-wrapped packaging.

takes several weeks. Haylage has gained popularity as an alternative to dry hay due to its low dust and mold levels, as well as its comparable or superior nutritive quality compared to dry hay (Séguin et al., 2010, 2012). Originally, haylage referred to silage with a DM content of approximately 50%. Nowadays, haylage is typically harvested at later growth stages, similar to hay, but baled before becoming completely dry, resulting in DM contents typically ranging from >50% to <70%, but occasionally up to 85% (Harris et al., 2017). However, a high moisture content in baled haylage, caused by unsuitable weather conditions during cutting and insufficient wilting or turning, can lead to the development of fungal spores and bacteria, increasing the risk of mycotoxin formation. Therefore, proper preservation under controlled conditions is necessary for forage (Harris et al., 2017).

Silage: Silage, on the other hand, is forage that is stored in an airtight environment with a DM content of less than 50%. In the process of silage production, water-soluble carbohydrates in the forage are fermented by anaerobic lactic acid bacteria, either naturally occurring on the crop or added as inoculants (Harris et al., 2017). To ensure sufficient lactic acid production during fermentation, the DM content of the crop should be around 30% or less (Harris et al., 2017). The preservation of silage occurs through fermentation, which progresses in three stages:

- **Phase I** is the aerobic (O_2) phase.
- **Phase II** is anaerobic, with increased anaerobic bacteria and lactic acid production. If not enough lactic acid is produced during this phase, butyric acid will be the more prevalent acid, causing odor, amino acid and protein breakdown, and decreased palatability.
- **Phase III** is a stable phase with a pH ≤ 4.5, which prevents the growth of spoilage microorganisms.

Straw: Straw, with its low energy and NSC content, can be considered as a forage option suitable for horses with low energy requirements. Previous studies indicated an increased risk of gastric ulcers when straw was provided as the sole source of forage, possibly related to lower intakes. However, recent research suggests that high-quality wheat straw, up to 50% of the forage diet, does not increase the risk of gastric ulcers and may even have positive effects on feeding behaviors and metabolic profiles, especially in overweight horses (Jansson et al., 2021). Untreated as well as ammoniated wheat straws have been found to be acceptable to horses when included at a 50% level in the forage diet (Hansen et al., 1992).

The slower consumption rate of straw compared to hay and cereals can increase the total daily eating time when straw is included in the diet (Meyer et al., 1975). This extended feeding time may contribute to increased satiety and potentially improved welfare for leisure or obese horses. Chewing activities in humans have been linked to reduced hunger levels and the activation of serotonin neurons in the brain, leading to suppressed feeding. This mechanism may also apply to horses, providing a possible explanation for the lower feed intake and increased ingestion breaks observed when horses are on a straw diet (Jansson et al., 2021).

It is important to note that the quality of straw is crucial, and good hygienic quality wheat, barley, or oaten straw should be selected for inclusion in the diet. Straw has a higher lignin and silica content than hay and will have lower digestibility. Incorporating straw into the ration can be a way to address the energy-restriction needs of horses while promoting natural feeding patterns and potential benefits to their metabolic profiles.

Forage analysis

Forage analysis is a valuable tool in assessing the contribution of forage to a horse's overall diet. Analyzing the nutritional composition of forage helps determine if the forage source is appropriate for the horse and if additional supplementation is necessary to meet nutritional requirements. Accredited laboratories specialize in testing the quality and nutritional value of forages for horses.

There are various types of forage analysis tests available:

- **NIR (near-infrared reflectance):** This test provides a basic analysis of the forage, including measurements of DM, CP, oil, ash, NDF, ADF, lignin, starch, sugar, and digestible energy. NIR is less accurate than wet chemistry but is a more cost-effective option. Some NIR assays also include mineral levels; however, accuracy is lower than with wet chemistry.
- **Wet chemistry:** This is a more appropriate analysis technique to use for soaked hays or forages that are not conserved. Wet chemistry analysis provides fundamental data on various parameters, including DM, CP, oil, ash, NDF, ADF, lignin, starch, sugar, and digestible energy. Wet chemistry can also include macro and trace minerals.
- **NSC analysis:** This is a method for quantifying and analyzing the levels of NSC in plants, which include sugars (such as glucose, fructose, and sucrose) and starch. This test is particularly useful for determining the suitability of the forage for horses with risks of conditions such as laminitis or metabolic syndrome.
- **Mineral analysis:** Forage analysis can also provide information about the mineral content of the forage. This includes measurements of minerals such as macro minerals calcium, phosphorus, magnesium, sodium, potassium, and chloride, as well as DCAB (dietary cation-anion balance) and trace mineral analysis. This analysis is useful in determining the need for added minerals in a forage-based diet.

By conducting forage analysis, horse owners and nutritionists can make informed decisions about the horse's diet, ensuring that the forage meets the necessary nutritional requirements and supports the horse's health and well-being.

Why and how should forages be soaked for horses?

Soaking forages in water before feeding has become a widely adopted practice in equine feeding (Figure 2.6). It serves various purposes, such as reducing the presence of respirable particles like mold spores and decreasing the content of NSC, energy, and some minerals.

Soaking hay is a common practice used to reduce the NSC and DE content in the forage in horse practices (Bochnia et al., 2021). The effectiveness of soaking depends on several factors, including time, temperature, volume of water, and rinsing. Studies have shown that soaking hay for 30 minutes can lead to a significant reduction of up to 90% in respirable particles, providing benefits for respiratory health (Müller et al., 2015). However, prolonged soaking does not result in any significant additional reduction in respirable particles (Moore-Colyer, 1996). On the other hand, soaking hay for 24 hours has been found to compromise the hygienic quality of the forage, as it increases the counts of yeast, lactic acid bacteria, and enterobacteria (Müller et al., 2015).

Overall, soaking forages can be an effective strategy for reducing respiratory risks associated with dust and mold spores, but it should be done within appropriate timeframes to maintain the hygienic quality of the forage (Martinson et al., 2012). Hay steamers can also be used for this purpose and can also improve the palatability of very dry hay.

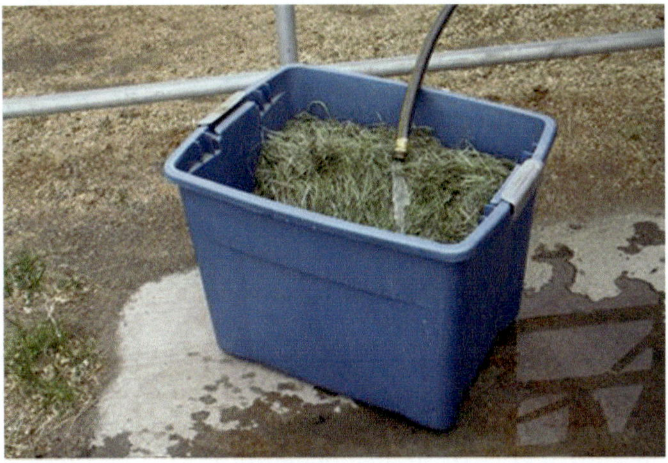

Figure 2.6 The soaking hay in a bucket.

Forage hygienic quality

Ensuring the hygienic quality of forages fed to horses is a critical concern due to the potential health risks associated with poor-quality forages. Poor hygienic quality in forages can result in a range of problems, such as the presence of dust, mold, mycotoxins, or bacterial contamination. For example, exposure to mold spores like *Aspergillus fumigatus* has been associated with recurrent airway obstruction in horses (Pirie, 2014). Additionally, botulinum toxin is a highly potent neurotoxin produced by the bacterium *Clostridium botulinum*, and its ingestion can lead to a severe condition known as botulism. This condition may manifest with symptoms such as muscle weakness and paralysis, and often results in death.

Feed hygiene, as outlined in EU legislation (Regulation (EC) No 183/2005), encompasses all aspects involved in producing, selling, and feeding safe feedstuff that does not pose any harmful effects to animals, including forages. The legislation (EC No 32/2002) sets maximum acceptable levels for various contaminants in feedstuffs, including heavy metals, aflatoxin B1, rye ergot, and pesticides, which are also applicable to forages.

Experts suggest that several parameters be considered when evaluating the hygienic quality of forages (Intemann et al., 2022; Wolf et al., 2014). These parameters help ensure that the forages meet the necessary safety standards and do not pose risks to the health and well-being of horses.

- **Macroscopic evaluation:** The primary method for assessing the hygienic quality of feedstuffs is through a macroscopic examination, although it is important to note that this test is subjective, and results may not be directly comparable between different individuals. However, clear criteria for evaluating feedstuffs provide a basis for approximate classification of hygienic quality (Kamphues et al., 2004). The macroscopic evaluation involves assessing various aspects such as the texture (e.g., dry or clammy), odor (e.g., typical, dusty or moldy), and color (e.g., green or bleached), and identifying any visible contaminants (e.g., sand, soil, or dead animals). It is recommended to regularly conduct macroscopic evaluations to identify obvious signs of mold as well as the presence of potentially harmful contaminants like sand, soil, and toxic plants such as *Senecio* spp. and *Taxus baccata* (Berny et al., 2010). This process helps determine the overall hygienic quality of the feedstuff and ensures that potential hazards are identified and addressed appropriately.
- **Microbiological evaluation:** Considerable attention is dedicated to the microbiological analysis of feedstuffs; however, it is important to acknowledge that the choice of analytical methods employed can significantly impact the results obtained. In certain European countries, there has been standardization in characterizing and establishing benchmarks for bacteria, molds, and yeasts in feedstuffs. These

benchmarks define the upper acceptable levels of contamination, which are believed to have no detrimental effects on the health of horses. Microorganisms found in feedstuffs are categorized as either epiphytic, meaning they are normal contaminants present even under optimal conditions, or spoilage-inducing. It is worth noting that both types of microorganisms can have health implications. It is crucial to highlight that while these benchmark levels serve as indicators of spoilage, a comprehensive assessment is necessary to determine the potential impact on equine health when these levels are exceeded (Harris et al., 2017). Under unfavorable conditions such as rain, high humidity, and elevated temperatures; undesirable bacteria, molds, and yeasts can proliferate in feedstuffs. However, it has been observed that a DM content exceeding 86% inhibits microbial and fungal activity. By drying hay to a DM content of over 86%, storage stability can be achieved. This indicates that hay, when sufficiently dried, can prevent the growth of microorganisms during storage due to the reduction in moisture content, which hinders their development (Kamphues et al., 2004). Hay that is baled with too much moisture can become warm and even spontaneously combust. The hay quality benchmark for yeast is 10^4 CFU/g, for mold is 70 x 10^3 CFU/g, and for bacteria is 10^6 CFU/g (Kamphues et al., 2004).

Mycotoxins

Mycotoxins are chemical compounds produced by molds that can be generated while cereals or forages are growing or being stored, and they have the potential to cause toxicity. Currently, approximately 300 mycotoxins have been identified, but there are likely many more yet to be discovered in nature. These mycotoxins tend to thrive in warm and humid environments, which makes tropical regions particularly vulnerable to their reproduction. Despite this knowledge, there is limited understanding regarding the impact of mycotoxins on the health of horses.

Some molds and mycotoxins mentioned earlier are typically present in or on plants before they are harvested. However, it is important to note that mycotoxin production may continue even after the harvest process. Another category of molds is known as storage molds (Figure 2.7). These molds typically contaminate animal feeds after harvest, although they can occasionally be found prior to harvesting as well. They are commonly observed on hay, silage, or grains that have been exposed to moisture or oxygen, usually due to inadequate packaging or improper storage conditions. Proper storage of forage and grains with low DM is crucial to prevent the growth of molds.

The European Food Safety Authority (EFSA) has taken steps to classify various mycotoxins as "undesirable substances in animal feed" in recent times. This classification is primarily intended to provide guidance values

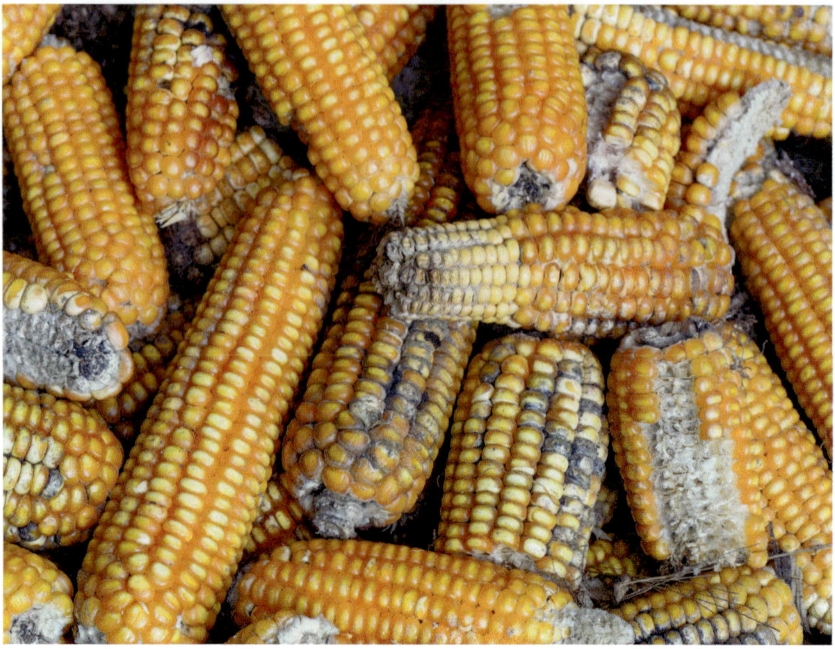

Figure 2.7 Image of mold growth and mycotoxins in corn during storage.

for the feed industry. While several mycotoxins have been identified as undesirable substances with maximum levels in human food, only aflatoxin B1 and rye ergot are currently recognized as such in animal feedstuffs. Among the mycotoxins commonly detected in horse feed are:

Aflatoxin: Aflatoxins are a group of mycotoxins primarily synthesized by *Aspergillus flavus* and *A. parasiticus*, which naturally contaminate food and feed. The main aflatoxins are B_1 (AFB_1), B_2 (AFB_2), G_1 (AFG_1), and G_2 (AFG_2), each exhibiting a distinct fluorescence color (B, blue; G, green) when exposed to ultraviolet light. *A. flavus* predominantly produces AFB_1 and AFB_2. Aflatoxin B1, classified as the most potent hepatocarcinogen by the International Agency for Research on Cancer (WHO, 1993), is a primary concern. Aflatoxin, a mycotoxin mainly generated by *Aspergillus* species, can be found in peanuts, soybeans, maize, copra meal, and other feed items.

The production of aflatoxin is highest at temperatures ranging from 25°C to 30°C and humidity levels of 97%–99%, which occurs mostly in tropical and subtropical regions. In horses, as well as other animal species, the liver is the target organ of aflatoxicosis. Horses affected by aflatoxin exposure display symptoms such as reduced feed intake, weight loss, neuro signs, and decreased productivity, which can significantly impact their athletic performance (Fink-Gremmels, 2008). There has been a suggested link between aflatoxin exposure and equine asthma (chronic obstructive pulmonary disease). Clinical changes and liver damage have been observed with a total dietary concentration of 500–1000 µg/kg (parts per billion), depending on the duration of exposure (Meerdink, 2002). Levels in feeds should be no greater than 20 parts per billion. This is an FDA limit.

Trichothecene deoxynivalenol: The trichothecenes are a group of epoxysesquiterpene metabolites produced by various fungal species belonging to the *Fusarium* genus, including *Fusarium graminearum*, *Fusarium sambucinum*, *Fusarium poae*, *Fusarium sporotrichioides*, and *Fusarium culmorum* (Desjardins et al., 1993). One prominent mycotoxin produced by these fungi is deoxynivalenol (DON), also known as vomitoxin, which can be found in different cereal crops. Corn and small grains are particularly susceptible to contamination by DON, making it the most prevalent mycotoxin in these crops. While DON exhibits toxic effects in all species, horses generally display greater tolerance compared to pigs (EFSA, 2004a). The major impact on horses is reduced palatability and feed intake.

Contaminated cereal grains such as corn, wheat, rye, barley, and oats are the primary sources of trichothecenes. The production of trichothecenes is influenced by high temperatures and high humidity. Among the trichothecenes, DON is often considered an indicator for the presence of other mycotoxins, as it remains relatively stable during drying, heating, and milling processes (Rotter et al., 1996). Limited data is available regarding DON contamination in forage, although it can be assumed that straw derived from contaminated grains may also be affected. Currently, EFSA guidance is that horse feeds should contain less than 3.5 ppm.

Zearalenone: Zearalenone, commonly referred to as ZEN, is a mycotoxin produced by various *Fusarium* species, including *F. roseum*, *F. tricinctum*, *F. sporotrichioides*, *F. oxysporum*, and *F. moniliforme* (Ropejko & Twarużek, 2021). These fungal species naturally occur in crops such as corn, barley, hay, oats, sesame, and sorghum. The presence of high humidity and low temperatures promotes the natural occurrence of ZEN.

In horses, ZEN induces estrogenic effects and is known to cause reproductive disorders (Gimeno & Quintavilla, 1983) and digestive disorders such as colic (Dänicke et al., 2021). Affected mares exhibited symptoms including feed refusal, swollen and edematous vulva, prolapsed vagina, enlarged uterus, and internal hemorrhage. Male horses displayed significant flaccidity of the genital organs.

Fumonisin: Fumonisins are mycotoxins produced by *Fusarium* species, specifically *Fusarium verticillioides* and *Fusarium proliferatum*. They naturally contaminate cereals, particularly corn and corn-based products. Three main types of fumonisin mycotoxins, namely fumonisin B1 (FB1), FB2, and FB3, have been found to occur naturally and at significant levels in corn as well as various animal feeds and human food items in several countries worldwide. Among domestic animals, horses are particularly susceptible to the toxic effects of FB1. When horses consume large quantities of corn infected with fumonisin, FB1 exhibits species-specific toxicity (Kellerman et al., 1990). The central nervous system, liver, and heart are the target organs in horses. Two distinct syndromes caused by FB1 toxicity have been identified: leukoencephalomalacia (ELEM), which is the neurotoxic form, and the hepatotoxic form. The neurotoxic form (ELEM) typically has a short clinical course, with the onset of acute signs followed by rapid death within hours or days. Mortality rates are usually high, and in some cases, death may occur without evident clinical signs. The hepatotoxic syndrome, on the other hand, occurs less frequently than the neurotoxic form and usually takes 5–10 days from the onset of clinical signs until death. The lowest observed adverse effect level is reported to be 0.2 mg/kg of BW or 2 ppm (EFSA, 2004b).

Ochratoxin A (OTA): OTA is a mycotoxin produced by various fungi belonging to the *Aspergillus* and *Penicillium* genera. In temperate climates, it is mainly produced by *P. verrucosum*, while in warm regions, *A. ochraceus* is the primary producer. Among animal feed materials, cereals are the most common sources of OTA contamination. Oats and wheat, along with their by-products like bran, pose the highest risks of contamination. A recent study found that 42% of horse feed grains were contaminated with OTA, with levels ranging from 0.2 to 4 µg/kg (Liesener et al., 2010). The kidneys are the target organs affected by ochratoxins. OTA is classified as a renal mycotoxin and a transplacental genotoxic carcinogen. Horses, being herbivores that rely on cecal fermentation rather than ruminal fermentation, have the potential to absorb OTA in the small intestine. It has been observed that OTA naturally occurs in horse serum samples and can be transferred through the placenta in horses (Minervini et al., 2013). Consequently, horses may be more sensitive to OTA toxicity than ruminants (EFSA, 2004c).

Although it is not feasible to completely eliminate mycotoxins, it is crucial to minimize contamination by improving harvesting and storage conditions. To ensure better control, additional analyses, including comprehensive assessments of mycotoxin levels, may be necessary.

Ergot alkaloids: Horses exhibit sensitivity to ergot alkaloids, particularly ergovaline, which can be found in pasture grasses infected with *Neotyphodium* spp. endophytes. The condition known as equine fescue toxicosis, primarily prevalent in the US, is caused by the consumption of endophyte-infected tall fescue (Figure 2.8). It is important to note that the effects of tall fescue on horses differ from those on other animals. In pregnant mares, fescue toxicosis can manifest through various clinical signs, including prolonged gestation, abortion, weakness, dysmaturity, mortality, thickened or retained placentas, and reduced lactation or agalactia. To mitigate these symptoms and minimize negative impacts on the reproductive system, removing pregnant mares from pastures infected

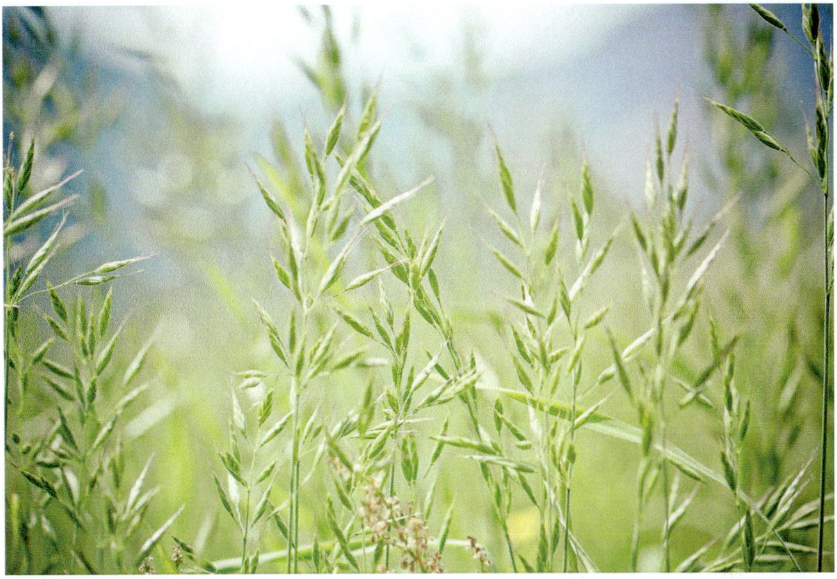

Figure 2.8 The meadow grass tall fescue (*Festuca partensis*) in spring.

with endophyte-infected tall fescue approximately 60 to 90 days before the expected foaling date is recommended (Evans, 2002). This allows the mare's body sufficient time to recover from any potential mycotoxin contamination prior to foaling. To minimize the risk of ergot alkaloid exposure, ensuring that horse feed contains no more than 5% rye is suggested, as rye is considered to be the cereal most susceptible to ergot contamination (EFSA, 2005a).

Botulinum: Botulism is an often fatal condition caused by the toxins produced by the anaerobic, spore-forming bacterium *Clostridium botulinum*, as well as other clostridia that produce botulinum toxins (including eight different serotypes). In adult horses, food-borne botulism occurs when they ingest preformed toxins, primarily of type B, C, or A. While outbreaks associated with hay or silage or alfalfa have been reported (Johnson et al., 2010; Wichtel & Whitlock, 1991), incidents of botulism in horses, mules, or cattle have frequently been linked to the consumption of big bale silage or haylage (Myllykoski et al., 2009). The production of botulinum toxin is typically triggered by contamination from animals, soil, or poultry slurry, including the incorporation of dead rodents or rabbits into hay, silage, or haylage. The utilization of waste obtained from anaerobic digesters in biogas production as fertilizer raises the likelihood of *C. botulinum* spore contamination in silage or haylage (Neuhaus et al., 2015).

Rhytisma: *Rhytisma acerinum* is a plant pathogen that primarily affects sycamore and maple trees during the summer and autumn seasons (Figure 2.9).

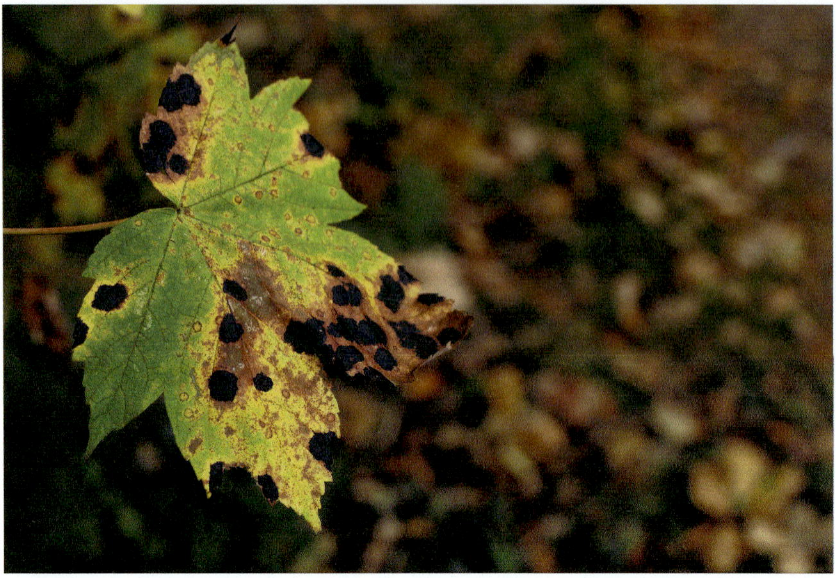

Figure 2.9 Rhytisma acerinum appears on maple leaves as black dots.

The visual appearance of the affected areas resembles the effect of tar droplets on leaves, which has led to the common name of "tar spots" for this disease. While tar spots is not generally considered to be highly detrimental to the trees, it can cause a condition called multiple acyl-CoA dehydrogenase deficiency, also known as atypical myopathy (AM), in horses that consume infected maple leaves (Van der Kolk, 2010). Maples belong to the Sapindaceae family, which is commonly referred to as the soapberry family. This plant family also includes other species like the horse chestnut. Within maple seeds, a chemical called hypoglycin A (2S-2-amino-3-(2-met hylidenecyclopropyl)-propanoic acid) is suspected of causing myopathies. Once ingested and metabolically activated, hypoglycin A transforms into a potent inhibitor of acyl-CoA dehydrogenase, a crucial enzyme involved in fatty acid metabolism (Gillman et al., 2014). Hypoglycin A can be detected in the blood of horses, but there are no detectable clinical signs in pastures where there is *A. pseudoplatanus* (sycamore maple). In spring, seedlings are a source of hypoglycin A intoxication; however, the disease is more prevalent in the autumn. Determination of hypoglycin A concentration in blood is useful for screening for exposure in suspected cases of AM (Baise et al., 2016). Populations of *Acer* that may contain hypoglycin A are present throughout the UK, US, and Europe and can be considered almost ubiquitous.

Practical advice for selecting forage for horses

A. The general recommendation for DM content in forage, according to Harris et al. (2017), is as follows:
   - For hay intended for forage, it is preferable to have a DM content of at least 86% or higher.
   - For haylage, which is forage stored in an airtight manner, the recommended DM content is 50% or higher.
   - Silage, also stored airtight, should have a DM content below 50%.

B. It is highly advisable to conduct a nutrient analysis of forage. This is particularly important when feeding horses with health issues such as gastric ulcers, poor body condition, obesity, pituitary pars intermedia dysfunction (PPID), laminitis, and polysaccharide storage myopathy (PSSM).

C. The hygienic quality of forages should be evaluated at both macro and micro levels. Poor hygienic quality can lead to significant health problems, including colic. It is essential to consider benchmarks for microorganism contamination to ensure proper quality control.

2.2 Concentrate feed

Concentrate is utilized either as a substitute for or in conjunction with forage blends to enhance energy density and supply essential nutrients to horses (Varloud et al., 2004). Straight grains like oats, corn, or barley have traditionally been employed to provide additional energy to specific types of horses, including racehorses (Richards et al., 2006) and show horses (Verhaar, 2010). In terms of horse feed, the consumption lies in complementary feedstuffs, predominantly cereal-based formulated feeds like "muesli," mash, extruded feeds, and pellets. Among the single-grain cereal feeds, oats, maize, and barley hold the most importance, and these vary depending on the country and type of the horse. These grains are utilized as sources of energy, principally from carbohydrates.

Fiber in feedstuffs

Oats have the highest fiber content among cereals, followed by barley, wheat, maize, and rice (NRC, 2007). The fiber content in oats is high primarily due to the presence of hulls, which contain a significant amount of NDF and ADF. These hulls consist of cellulose and xylan, which are much less digestible than the starch found in the oat kernel, thus reducing the energy content of oats. Some oat varieties have a lower lignin content in their hulls, and consequently, they are more digestible. In contrast, naked oats, which are free of hulls, have higher fat content (12%–15%) and higher starch content and, therefore, provide more energy than regular oats.

Not only does the fiber content differ among cereals, but the quality of the fiber also varies. Oats and barley, for example, contain β-glucans in their fiber fraction, while wheat, rye, and triticale contain arabinoxylans (Knudsen, 1997). Both soluble β-glucans and arabinoxylans have viscous properties that can influence the gut environment and potentially affect digestive processes. Diets with high inclusion of oats and barley (rich in soluble β-glucans) or wheat, rye, and triticale (rich in soluble arabinoxylans) may contribute to disruptions in gut function (Geor et al., 2013). However, this may be less of a concern in diets where the main cereal sources are maize (corn) or rice, as they contain low levels of both soluble β-glucans and arabinoxylans (Geor et al., 2013). However, they also contain less fiber and more starch than grains like oats, making them less safe to feed.

Super fibers: Feeding sugar beet pulp or soybean hulls, both of which are highly digestible and referred to as super fibers, can also increase fiber intake. Compared with more traditional fiber sources such as hay, soybean hulls, and beet pulp contain lower levels of indigestible material (e.g., lignin, silica) and higher amounts of hemicellulose, NSPs, pectins, and gums, which can be digested to a large extent within the time that they remain in the gastrointestinal tract. This translates to a higher energy yield.

- **Sugar beet pulp:** Beet pulp is the readily digestible fiber that remains once sugar has been extracted from sugar beets. Sugar beet pulp can serve as an alternative to hay as a forage source in the diet without compromising hindgut function (Hyslop et al., 1997). This makes it an affordable feed choice that is relatively high in pectin and other soluble fibers. The breakdown of beet pulp in the horse's digestive system depends on microbial fermentation in the hindgut. When molasses is added to beet pulp, it increases the sugar and glycemic index (GI) of the feed, while some commercial beet pulp products are processed to be low in sugar. It is often recommended to soak beet pulp in water before feeding, especially when feeding larger amounts (>0.5 kg), to improve palatability and reduce the risk of esophageal obstruction due to dry feed impaction. Soaking and rinsing can also reduce the sugar content and lower the GI of the beet pulp. Additionally, beet pulp has a higher water-holding capacity than hay or soybean hulls. It is often used as a component or included in mixed feeds.
- **Soybean hulls:** Soybean hulls have been a staple in horse nutrition for many years, primarily serving as a valuable source of dietary fiber. They are among the most commonly utilized super fibers in horse diets. Soybean hulls are notable for their high hemicellulose level, fermentable fiber, and high fiber digestibility. While they have low levels of NSCs (sugars and starches), they contain fiber that is highly digestible for horses. The NDF and ADF concentrations in soybean hulls are similar to hay, making them a practical addition to the diet. However,

it is recommended to limit the inclusion of soybean hulls to less than 50% of the diet. When high amounts of soybean hulls were combined with alfalfa in quarter horses, it led to an increase in VFA propionate and a decrease in cecal pH (Coverdale et al., 2004). Additionally, soybean hulls could replace up to 75% of traditional alfalfa-brome grass hay without compromising acceptability (Coverdale et al., 2004). Furthermore, soybean hulls are commonly employed as carriers for supplements in the equine industry.

It is reasonable to substitute 15% of the energy in the diet of a performance horse with highly fermentable fiber. However, this may not provide the same performance benefits as adding 15% of the energy from oil in the diet (Crandell et al., 1999).

Starch and sugar in feedstuffs

Starch is composed of glucose polymers and exists in two forms: amylose and amylopectin. Amylose is a linear molecule linked by α-(1–4) bonds, while amylopectin is a larger molecule with extensive branching, containing both α-(1–4) and α-(1–6) linkages (Geor et al., 2013).

Starch is a highly digestible energy source that plays a vital role in meeting the energy requirements of horses for various physiological functions, growth, and exercise. It is primarily broken down by the enzyme amylase in the small intestine during digestion, producing glucose, which is essential for the body's metabolic processes. The digestion of starch is influenced by factors such as intake level, origin, and feed processing methods. Among commonly used cereals, rice has the highest starch content, followed by maize, wheat, barley, and oats in descending order (NRC, 2007). However, when oats are de-hulled, there is a significant increase in the starch content and a noticeable decrease in fiber content, making the carbohydrate composition comparable to that of barley (Knudsen, 1997). De-hulling oats improves fat content and nutrient digestibility, and leads to a higher energy value for horses.

The proportion of amylose and amylopectin in starch varies depending on its botanical source. For example, wheat flour contains approximately 30% amylose, while maize can contain up to 70% amylose. Furthermore, starch molecular weight can vary significantly, which may impact digestibility. Glucose availability tends to be higher with amylopectin-type starch (Geor et al., 2013). Not all grains have equal starch digestibility in a horse's small intestine, and while oat starch is well digested, other grains such as barley, corn, and wheat require heating to gelatinize starch and increase digestibility (Meyer et al., 1986). The heat can come from boiling, steam flaking, extruding, or micronizing. Undigested starch from rolled or cracked grain that has not been heated can contribute to hindgut acidosis and significant disturbances of the microbiota.

Sport horses, which have high energy demands, are typically provided with concentrated feeds that are rich in energy and contain a significant amount of starch. However, it is important to feed starch in appropriate amounts to avoid potential health issues. When horses consume excess starch that cannot be digested in the small intestine, it passes through to the large intestine, where it undergoes fermentation to produce energy. However, excessive starch in the large intestine can lead to health problems such as a decrease in colon and/or cecal pH, which may result in conditions like colic, laminitis, or hindgut acidosis. Hindgut lactic acidosis can occur due to increased acidity in the hindgut. The influence of different levels of dietary starch on glycogen restoration in working horses was investigated. Studies (Pagan et al., 2015; Stewart et al., 2017) found that high starch intake resulted in more effective glycogen replenishment compared to moderate or low starch consumption in these horses. Notably, a minor decrease in glycogen levels after exercise in horses with moderate and low starch diets suggested that fat or protein might have been utilized as an energy source during physical activity. The research outcomes indicated that supplying 1.2 g/kg BW of starch per day did not offer any recovery time advantage over a moderate- or low-starch diet in light-working horses; however, it may be required in harder-working horses where greater glycogen depletion occurs. Therefore, while starch is necessary in a horse's diet, it is crucial to ensure it is fed in appropriate quantities to maintain digestive health and prevent potential complications.

Molasses, derived from beet and cane, and syrup made from hydrolyzed starch are the most commonly used types of sugar in equine diets. Horses efficiently utilize simple sugars such as glucose and fructose, which are easily absorbed in the small intestine. Similarly, hydrolyzed starch, consisting of glucose, maltose, and maltotriose, is digested and utilized well by horses.

However, there are limitations to the digestive capacity of certain disaccharides, depending on the age of the horse and changes in the secretion of digestive enzymes (Meyer, 1992). Foals, with their high activity of lactase, effectively utilize lactose, while their ability to utilize sucrose is less efficient due to their limited activity of sucrase. In contrast, adult horses exhibit the reverse pattern. Meyer (1992) suggests that the maximum dietary inclusion of lactose in adult horses should not exceed 1 g/kg of BW per day to prevent digestive disturbances. It is commonly recommended to use molasses in the equine diet at a concentration of less than 10% of the concentrate portion. As the majority of horse feeds or diets typically include only limited quantities of molasses, this isn't a significant concern for horses.

There are advantages and disadvantages associated with the use of molasses in equine diets.

Advantages:

- Highly palatable, enhancing the overall taste and appeal of the diet.
- Plays a role in reducing dust, creating a cleaner feeding environment by minimizing airborne particles.
- Helps in binding mixed feed ingredients together, promoting cohesion and ensuring that the components stay well-integrated.

Disadvantages:

- Increases NSC content in feed.
- Rapid intake leads to a higher GI.
- Contains a high potassium content, typically ranging from 4% to 5% potassium (K).

Fructan

Fructan is a significant complex carbohydrate found in equine diets. Unlike simple sugars and starches, fructan is classified as an NSC but is not digested in the small intestine and, like other fiber-based complex carbohydrates, requires fermentation in the hindgut. Fructan is a type of carbohydrate that plants store as an energy source, and it is found in higher concentrations in cool-season grasses like timothy, orchard grass, brome, and ryegrass, as well as the hay made from them. The fructan content of pasture grass can increase due to a variety of environmental factors.

Non-fiber carbohydrate = 100% – (Crude protein % + Neutral detergent fiber % + Moisture % + Crude fat % + Crude ash %)

Non-structural carbohydrate = starch + water-soluble carbohydrate

Fructan = Water-soluble carbohydrate – Ethanol-soluble carbohydrate

A high amount of fructan or an overload of starch will each result in a change in gastrointestinal flora, reduced intestinal pH, and increased permeability, and as a consequence, absorption of laminitis-triggering factors such as bacterial exotoxins, endotoxins, and vasoactive amines (Geor, 2010). Therefore, it is recommended to limit starch intake to no more than 1.1 g/kg of BW per meal and to opt for forage containing less than 10% NSC, especially in specific cases like horses prone to PSSM or laminitis (Geor, 2010).

Protein in feedstuffs

Canola meal, soybean meal, linseed meal, cottonseed meal, lupins, peas, beans, sunflower seeds or meal, and dried brewer's grain are widely used

Table 2.3 The average crude protein (CP) content and amino acid content of common protein sources on an as-fed basis

Feed types	*% Dry matter*	*% CP (as-fed basis)*	*% Lysine (as-fed basis)*	*% Methionine (as-fed basis)*	*% Threonine (as-fed basis)*
Soybean meal*	89	42.3	2.9	0.7	1.8
Canola meal	90	32.0	2.1	0.7	1.6
Linseed meal	90	30.2	1.2	0.6	1.1
Sunflower meal*	93	39.2	1.2	0.8	1.4
Cottonseed meal	90	37.2	1.7	0.7	1.3

Source: Adapted from NRC 2007, page 164
* *Soybean meal and sunflower meal are hull-free.*

as protein-rich feedstuffs in horse diets (Table 2.3). The levels of CP and amino acid content differ depending on the feeds.

- Soybean meal is an excellent protein source for horses due to its high-quality amino acid composition and protein content ranging from 43% to 50% (NRC). Specifically, it is abundant in essential amino acids like lysine, which is considered the "first limiting" amino acid, as well as methionine and threonine. Because of these qualities, many premium commercial horse feed formulations incorporate soybean meal as a key ingredient. Whole soybeans need to undergo processes like roasting or extrusion to inactivate naturally occurring trypsin inhibitors, lectins, and saponins that can hinder protein digestion and act as antinutritional factors. These processes involve heating, which can destroy trypsin inhibitors in soybeans and peas, as well as deactivate toxins like gossypol found in cottonseed meal, thus making them suitable for inclusion in horse feeds. Full-fat soybean meal, produced through cooking or roasting soybeans, contains high fat levels and offers a rich source of all essential amino acids.
- Canola meal is a protein-rich by-product resulting from the extraction of oil from canola seeds. It closely matches the nutritional composition of soybean meal, although it contains less lysine. Canola used to be known as rapeseed and has some antinutritional factors, but modern varieties of canola meal are very safe to feed to horses.
- Linseed is often categorized among other "oilseeds," such as canola (a brassica) and soybeans (a legume). Historically, horse owners primarily fed linseed to horses in the form of a linseed mash, which became a highly favored protein supplement for horse nutrition. However, linseed has a low lysine content compared to other protein sources. Raw linseed contains an enzyme called linase, which, in moist conditions, has the potential to release hydrogen cyanide. Micronization and or heating not only enhances the nutritional value and taste but also

deactivates linase, making the resulting product suitable for direct feeding. One of the primary advantages of micronized linseed for horses is its rich content of omega-3 fatty acids.

- Cottonseed meal is what's left after the oil has been extracted from cotton seeds, and it's valued as a protein-rich animal feed. It is commonly used as a protein source for horses in some areas because of its wide availability and appealing taste. However, it is worth noting that cottonseed meal doesn't contain as much lysine as soybean or canola meal. Raw cottonseeds contain the antinutritional factor gossypol, which can inhibit protein digestion unless it is inactivated by heat.
- Sunflower meal, which is the by-product of sunflower seed oil extraction, boasts a substantial protein content. While it has lower protein content and significantly higher fiber content compared to soybean meal, sunflower meal remains a valuable option for feeding horses. Sunflower seeds are fed in some parts of the world as a palatable source of oil and protein.
- Legumes such as lupins, beans, and peas are also fed for protein and energy. They need to be cracked or cooked by steaming or micronizing and flaked. Some varieties contain anti-nutritional factors which need to be inactivated by processing.
- Among common cereals, wheat has the highest protein content, followed by oats and barley, while rice and maize have the lowest protein content. When assessing protein quality based on lysine content, oats, barley, and rice have higher protein quality compared to wheat and maize. Barley is intermediate between oats and corn in terms of CP and lysine levels. The proteins found in maize grain primarily consist of zein and glutelin. Zein, being the most significant, has deficiencies in lysine and tryptophan, requiring amino acid supplementation in equine diets. However, alternatives such as corn gluten feed, corn gluten meal, and corn distillers' grains may be preferable choices due to their higher protein and fiber content and lower starch content.
- Including urea in the diet of horses does not improve protein quality and can be toxic and fatal in high amounts. Therefore, its use in horse diets is not recommended.

Fat in feedstuffs

In terms of fat content, oats have higher levels compared to other grains, containing more than twice the amount of fat as barley, according to the National Research Council (2007) (as shown in Table 2.4). This difference is also reflected in the content of specific essential fatty acids such as linoleic and α-linolenic acid.

- In regular oats, fat contributes to approximately 10% of the DE content with 6% fat, 41% starch, and 9% CP. On the other hand, other

Table 2.4 Average nutrient composition of selected horse feedstuffs

Nutrient composition as fed	*Oat grain, rolled*	*Barley grain, rolled*	*Corn grain, cracked, dry*	*Wheat bran*	*Rice bran*	*Beet pulp, unmolassed*
DM %	90	91	88	89	90	88
DE MJ/kg as fed	12.3	13.9	14.3	11.9	12.6	10.3
CP % as fed	11.9	11.3	8.3	15.4	13.9	8.8
Lysine % as fed	0.5	0.41	0.24	0.6	0.6	0.4
Crude fat % as fed	4.6	2	3.7	3.8	13.7	0.9
NDF % as fed	27	18.9	8.4	37.8	23.5	40.3
ADF % as fed	13.1	6.6	3	13.8	11.8	20.3
Ash % as fed	3	2.6	1.3	5.6	9.36	6.4

Source: adapted from NRC 2007, page 304)

commonly used cereals in monogastric diets, such as wheat and rice, typically have fat contributing to approximately 3%–5% of the DE content.

- Rice bran has a similar NDF content to oats, but the NDF is highly digestible and has a higher fat content, ranging from 15% to 20%. This makes rice bran a valuable source of high-energy fat. However, the challenge with full-fat rice bran is the potential for rancidity during storage due to the presence of a lipolytic enzyme that becomes active when the bran is separated from the rice. Rice bran rancidity is particularly problematic in tropical areas. To overcome this issue, stabilized rice bran is a preferred option for horse feeding. Stabilized rice bran is processed soon after milling to inactivate the lipase enzyme, reducing the potential for rancidity.
- Other high-fat ingredients include sunflower seeds, which can be up to 40% fat, and roasted soybeans or full-fat soybeans, which can be 20% fat.

Minerals in feedstuffs

All grains are low in calcium, especially oats (1.2 g/kg DM), barley (0.7 g/kg DM), wheat (0.7 g/kg DM), and corn (0.4 g/kg DM) (Geor et al., 2013). By-products exhibit varying calcium levels, ranging from 2 g/kg DM in wheat bran to over 15 g/kg DM in citrus pulp (Geor et al., 2013). Barley and oats contain approximately 8 grams of phytate and 11 grams of total inositol phosphates per kg DM, which can form complexes with phosphorus, calcium, iron, and zinc (Brooks & Lampi, 2001). Wheat middlings and bran contain 1% phosphorus and 80% of this as phytates, resulting in an unbalanced calcium-to-phosphorus ratio. However, processing wheat bran into pellets can significantly reduce its phytate activity due to heat destruction.

Grain by-products

Grain by-products in horse feed are residual materials and substances derived from grain processing that are incorporated into equine diets to improve nutritional content and energy density. They are frequently included in horse feeds to add nutrients and energy, and the specific by-products used can vary depending on the formulation and nutritional needs of the horses being fed. Because of differences in processing techniques between mills, the nutritional makeup of by-product feeds is more inconsistent than that of whole grains. Nonetheless, these by-product feeds are frequently cost-effective and have a variety of nutritional qualities that make them suitable for horse feeding.

Wheat middlings (midds) are a common grain by-product used in horse feeds. Wheat midds are higher in fiber and protein than wheat grain, but lower in energy and starch because most of the flour has been removed. When using wheat midds in horse feed, the calcium-to-phosphorous ratio must be balanced with calcium supplementation to the diet. Wheat bran is also commonly used in horse feeds because it contains more ADF and NDF than wheat midds and is high in phosphorus. Most of the phosphorus in wheat midds and wheat bran is accounted for by phytate. Phytate, also known as phytic acid, is a compound found in plant seeds. It has the potential to reduce nutrient absorption.

Rice bran, which is commonly used in horse feed, contains roughly the same amount of NDF as oats but is relatively high in crude fat. Rice bran contains some non-fiber carbohydrates, including starch. When using rice bran in horses' diets, two important factors must be considered. The first is that rice bran may have an inverted calcium-to-phosphorous ratio, and the second is that rice bran may contain a naturally occurring lipase that certain types of processing can inactivate. As a result, stabilized rice bran is recommended for use because it reduces the potential for rancidity. Rice bran processed soon after milling to inactivate this lipase is called stabilized rice bran. The Association of American Feed Control Officials (AAFCO) (2005) states that the free fatty acid content of crude fat in rice bran must be less than 4%.

Corn gluten feed, corn gluten meal, and corn distillers' dried grains are by-products of corn processing or distillation. Compared to corn, these substances contain significantly more protein and fiber but significantly less starch. Therefore, it is frequently used in horse feed. Oats can be cleaned to remove loose hulls. Oat hulls have high levels of NDF and ADF, which can be used to increase dietary fiber content. Nonetheless, they have only limited digestibility in horses, which means they provide limited energy to equine diets.

Barley is the most commonly used grain in the brewing industry, and brewers frequently supply dried grains for animal feeds. Dried grains from brewers typically have higher protein and fiber content while containing less starch than whole grains.

Some by-products are not suitable for use in horses because the fiber is too indigestible (e.g., sugar cane bagasse, canola hulls, peanut hulls, sunflower hulls) or because of risks of mycotoxin contamination (e.g., peanut hulls).

2.3 Feed processing

Feed processing plays a significant role in the extent of prececal starch digestion in horses. Cereal grains like oats, barley, and corn are major sources of starch in horses' diets, and the composition of starch in these grains consists of amylose and amylopectin molecules. Starch digestion is affected by factors such as intake level, botanical origin, genotype, and feed processing methods. Processing grains using heat and moisture enhances the availability of starch for enzymatic degradation, leading to increased digestion in the small intestine. This enzymatic digestion in the small intestine is preferred over fermentation in the hindgut, as hindgut fermentation can result in higher concentrations of short-chain fatty acids and lactate, decreased pH, and disturbances in microbial balance in horses.

Concentrate feeds, a significant source of NSCs in equine diets, typically contain grains that contribute 30%–50% of NSC on an as-fed basis. However, many modern compounded feeds utilize grain by-products or forage products instead of grains, resulting in a lower overall NSC content. Pleasure horse feeds, on average, contain approximately 15%–30% of NSC on an as-fed basis, while specialty feeds can have NSC levels as low as 10%. Recent research has demonstrated that a concentrate feed containing 30% processed grains can improve digestion without adversely affecting feeding behavior or fecal pH (Kalantari et al., 2021).

Various techniques are employed to enhance the nutritional value of feeds by improving the availability and digestibility of starch (Table 2.5). Grains are often subjected to different processing methods, including mechanical processes such as rolling, crushing, cracking, and grinding, as well as thermal processes like roasting, pelleting, and micronizing. Additionally, thermo-mechanical approaches such as steam flaking, popping, and extruding are utilized. These processes can be carried out under dry or wet conditions involving steam, such as steam rolling, steam crushing, steam flaking, pressure toasting, steam extruding, expanding, and pelleting (Julliand et al., 2006). The effect of heat on increased pre-ileal

Table 2.5 Effect of processing corn on pre-ileal starch digestibility in horses

Feeds	*Apparent digestibility (%)*
Whole or cracked corn	29
Ground corn, modern mill	47
Expanded corn	90

Source: Kienzle et al., 1997

starch digestibility and GI is demonstrated in the table below and is also seen with barley. However, oat starch is well digested in the small intestine (>80%) without heating, and flaking/rolling only leads to a small increase in digestibility.

Processing can influence palatability and rate of intake, as well as digestibility. Pelleted and unprocessed grain feeds have been shown to have faster intake rates than extruded feeds. This is probably because extruded feeds are less dense, but it may also relate to particle size and shape. Large flaked or micronized grains such as corn or beans can also be slightly less palatable for some horses.

2.4 Fats

Numerous studies have investigated the impact of incorporating fat into the diet of performance horses (Potter et al., 1992; Pagan, 2020). These studies have observed changes in blood parameters during exercise when comparing diets with fat added to traditional grain-based rations 1995. In most of these studies, fat was used to replace a portion of the grain in the diet, reducing total starch intake. While it is reasonable to substitute 15% of the digestible energy in a performance horse's diet with a highly fermentable fiber, it may not offer the same performance advantages as adding 15% as vegetable oil (Crandell et al., 1999).

Fat-added feeds have generally been found to be palatable to horses, particularly when vegetable oils such as corn, soybean, sunflower, and flaxseed oil are used (Figure 2.10). Corn oil, in particular, has shown to be well accepted when incorporated into a diet (Holland et al., 1998). Horses readily accept diets containing up to 15% added corn oil (Holland et al., 1998). However, the acceptability of other types of fats has not been extensively studied and anecdotal evidence raises questions about their palatability when the fat sources age or are added in large amounts. Solid high-fat sources such as full-fat soy, stabilized rice bran, linseed, or sunflower seeds provide a more palatable way of providing fat-based energy to the horse.

Fatty acids are grouped based on the presence and number of double bonds in their carbon chain. Saturated fatty acids have no double bonds,

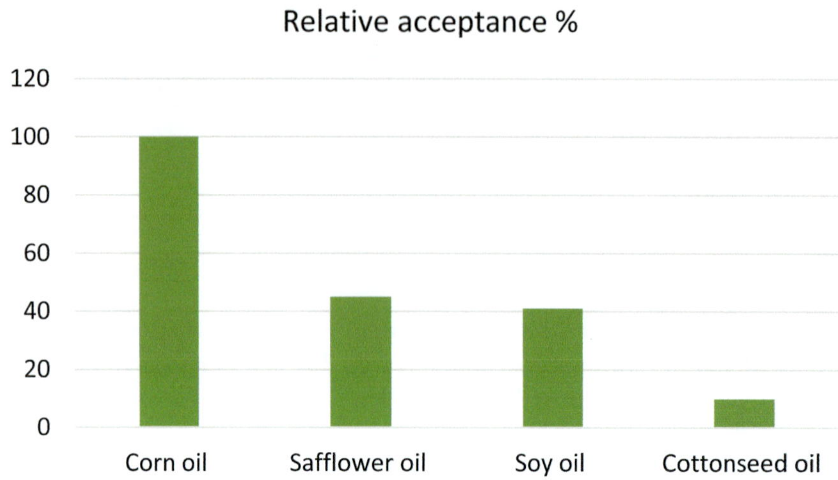

Figure 2.10 Relative acceptance of fats evaluated in palatability experiments compared to corn oil (adapted from Holland et al. 1998).

monounsaturated fatty acids (MUFAs) have one double bond, and polyunsaturated fatty acids (PUFAs) have more than one double bond. Based on the position of the initial double bond, unsaturated fatty acids can be further classified into three main families.

- **Omega-3 fatty acids** play a vital role in cell membrane function, and long-chain forms have anti-inflammatory properties. The primary omega-3 fatty acid is alpha-linolenic acid (ALA) and its long-chain derivatives, including eicosapentaenoic acid (EPA) and docosahexaenoic acid (DHA). Grass has a 3:1 ratio of omega-3 to omega-6 fatty acids. Flaxseed is a significant source of short-chain ALA (18:3 omega-3), while fish oil contains long-chain EPA (20:5 omega-3) and DHA (22:6 omega-3), which are the primary omega-3 fatty acids present.
- **Omega-6 fatty acids** play a crucial role in maintaining the integrity of cell membranes, promoting gastrointestinal health, and supporting immune and inflammatory functions (Mori & Hodgson, 2013). The main omega-6 fatty acid is linoleic acid (LA), and its derivative, arachidonic acid (AA), is also significant in these functions. Omega-6 fatty acids, including LA, are involved in various physiological processes in horses. They contribute to forming and maintaining healthy cell membranes, supporting skin and coat health, and playing a role in immune and inflammatory responses. One long-chain omega-6 fatty acid, DGLA (20:3 omega-6), has anti-inflammatory properties, but AA 20:4 is a pro-inflammatory mediator.

- **Omega-9 fatty acids** are primarily represented by oleic acid (18:1 ω9). Omega-9 fatty acids are classified as monounsaturated fatty acids. Oleic acid is commonly found in various dietary fat sources, including vegetable oils such as olive oil and canola oil. While omega-9 fatty acids are not essential for horses, they can still contribute to overall dietary fat composition. Including moderate amounts of omega-9 fatty acids in the equine diet through appropriate oil supplementation or natural sources can help provide a balanced fatty acid profile.

The essential fatty acids that horses need to obtain from their diet because their bodies cannot synthesize them are omega-3 and omega-6. The fatty acid profiles of common oil sources are displayed in Table 2.6. Flaxseed oil is a rich source of omega-3 fatty acids, in contrast to corn and soybean oils, which are sources of omega-6 series fatty acids. Dietary supplementation with omega-3 fatty acids has been associated with systemic anti-inflammatory effects in various species, resulting from alterations in AA metabolism and reduced production of pro-inflammatory substances.

Dietary supplementation with flaxseed oil has been shown to decrease the leukocyte response to inflammation in horses (Morris et al., 1991). Coconut oil and its derivative medium-chain triglyceride (MCT) oil have gained popularity as energy and wellness supplements in the equine industry. The palatability of corn oil versus MCT oil or coconut oil when mixed with concentrate feed is the same for horses. Horses, however, prefer concentrate without added oil over concentrate mixed with oil as excessive added oil can reduce palatability. The inclusion of fish oil in the diet has garnered attention as it has potential benefits for glucose tolerance (Huntington et al., 2013) and insulin sensitivity (Hess et al., 2013), although further research is needed for clarification of dose and time considerations. Portier et al. (2006) studied the effect of omega-3 on erythrocyte membrane fluidity (EMF) modulation in horses by giving 12 healthy, trained horses either an omega-3 supplement or a placebo for four weeks. All horses performed standardized exercise tests, and blood samples were collected throughout the trial. Omega-3 induced changes in membrane composition, which modulated the decrease in EMF induced by exercise. Omega-3 supplementation may be beneficial for sport horses in regular exercise. Feeding horses with fish oil significantly raised the levels of circulating EPA and DHA in plasma (King et al., 2008) and in tissues (Vineyard et al., 2010), whereas flaxseed oil did not increase the levels of the long-chain omega-3 fatty acids. Not surprisingly, the same effect was seen in a comparison of fish oil and corn oil (Huntington et al., 2010), and in general terms, if you are looking for an increase in tissue levels of the long-chain omega-3 fatty acids EPA and DHA, you need to feed fish oil for at least 30 days. Feeding flaxseed or flaxseed oil will not achieve the same effect.

Table 2.6 Fatty acid composition of different feed source types (g/kg DM)

Type of oil	*Linoleic acid (ω-6, 18:2n-6)*	*α-linolenic acid (ω-3, 18:2n-3)*	*EPA (20:5n-3)*	*DHA (22:6n-3)*
Corn oil	532	11	0	0
Soybean oil	504	67	0	0
Sunflower oil	287	0.4	0	0
Rice bran oil	71	3.2	0	0
Canola oil	186	91	0	0
Flaxseed oil	127	533	0	0
Fish oil (menhaden)	21	14	131	85
Fish oil, salmon	15	10	130	182
Grass hay, cool-season	2	4	0	0
Legume hay	3	4	0	0
Green grass	4	14	0	0
Barley grain	10	1.1	0	0
Oat grain	23	1	0	0
Soybean meal	10	1	0	0

Source: data adapted from the NRC, 2007 and Geor et al., 2013

Dietary omega-3 from fish oil modulates the inflammatory response of horses and should be considered in treating equine recurrent airway obstruction or other equine inflammatory diseases (Nogradi et al., 2015). An update study on exercise-induced pulmonary hemorrhage (EIPH) in horses (Poole & Erickson, 2016) supported using long-chain omega-3 supplementation from fish oil in decreasing EIPH occurrence and severity as a 143-day-long trial by Kansas State University had already concluded. Diets rich in DHA and EPA from fish oil can reduce EMF during exercise and improve pulmonary hemodynamics, reducing the severity of EIPH. While there is currently no strong evidence of effectiveness in horses, the potential utility of PUFAs in equine osteoarthritis has led to their incorporation in some oral joint supplements.

While there is no established ideal ratio for horses, it has been suggested that a higher omega-3 to omega-6 ratio in the diet can reduce inflammation and muscle damage after exercise (O'Connor et al., 2004).

Due to its importance in various biological processes, incorporating fat into the equine diet has been demonstrated to offer several additional advantages.

The inclusion of oil in a horse's diet offers advantages

- Reduces the dustiness of feed.
- Prevents the caking of sweet feeds.
- Improves feed preparation and enhances feed mixing quality.
- Acts as a binder and lubricant for pelleting.
- Promotes a glossy hair coat in horses.
- Increases the energy/caloric density of a meal.
- Serves as an alternative to starch (non-structural carbohydrates) as a dietary energy source.
- Reduces thermal load during exercise, benefiting the horse by reducing heat production.
- Supports the health and function of the gastrointestinal tract.
- Improves aerobic capacity, allowing horses to perform better during activities.
- Helps to stabilize temperament and reduce excitability or nervousness.
- Reduces the overall glycemic index of the feed.
- Reduces the likelihood of muscle fatigue and tying up due to providing a more sustainable source of energy.

The inclusion of oil in a horse's diet may have some potential disadvantages

- Digestive upset: Some horses may have difficulty digesting oil, especially if it is added in large quantities or introduced too quickly. Rapid changes in the diet can lead to digestive upset, such as diarrhea or colic.
- Palatability: Not all horses are willing to consume oil willingly.
- Imbalanced nutrition: While oil is a good source of calories, it lacks essential nutrients such as amino acids, vitamins, and minerals.
- Weight gain and obesity: Oil is calorie-dense, and excessive consumption without adequate exercise can lead to weight gain and obesity in horses.
- Slow glycogen repletion: Oil can lead to slow glycogen repletion in very high-fat diets fed to hard-working horses (Pagan et al., 2015).
- Oxidation and rancidity: Oil can become rancid when exposed to air, heat, and light. Rancid oil not only loses its nutritional value but can also be unappetizing and potentially harmful. It's crucial to store oil properly in cool, dark conditions and use it within its recommended shelf life.
- Cost: Oil costs more compared to other calorie sources.

Before adding oil to a horse's diet, it is advisable to consult with a veterinarian or equine nutritionist who can assess your horse's individual needs and provide specific recommendations. They can help determine the appropriate type, amount, and method of incorporating oil into the horse's diet while considering any potential disadvantages and monitoring the horse's response.

2.5 Supplements

- Supplements or "feed additives" are substances, microorganisms, or preparations intentionally added to feed or water to perform specific functions defined in Regulation (EC) No 1831/2003 of the European Parliament and of the Council of 22 September 2003 on additives for use in animal nutrition.
- In the UK and EU, the market for feed and supplement brands is diverse and fragmented, making it challenging for customers to choose. A study in New England showed that 84% of participants used at least one supplement on average in their horses' diets (Hoffman et al., 2009). A wide range of equine nutritional supplements is available in the UK, with approximately 171,400 purchases made annually (Agar et al., 2016).
- The Feed Additives Regulation of 2003 establishes a standardized procedure for authorizing feed additives and sets guidelines for their market placement, labeling, and usage. Horse owners consider various factors when selecting nutritional supplements for their horses, including discipline-specific health and performance concerns, as well as any pre-existing issues or injuries in individual animals (Williams et al., 2019).
- Practically, supplements are often used as feedstuffs that do not exceed 5% of the total ration's weight and do not include items like carrots, apples, or mints. These supplements can be categorized based on their core purpose (Harris & Dunnett, 2018).

Fundamental dietary supplements

These supplements typically contain substances that fulfill established nutritional requirements, including vitamins, minerals, trace elements, and amino acids (Harris & Dunnett, 2018), and often these are combined in high-protein vitamin and mineral balancer pellets.

Vitamin and mineral supplements: The National Research Council (NRC) has established the nutrient requirement values as minimum allowances for intakes of some vitamins and minerals in equine nutrition. However, this only covers a few B vitamins apart from B1 and B2 (NRC, 2007). Improper use of feed supplements can disrupt the natural balance of vitamins and minerals in a horse's diet. This can potentially lead to deficiencies in certain nutrients, although signs of deficiencies are uncommon. Instead, horses are more likely to risk receiving excessive levels of certain nutrients, which can be toxic. For instance, cobalt is a crucial micronutrient necessary for vitamin B12 synthesis in the equine cecum and colon. Normally, adult horses obtain an adequate amount of cobalt from their diet to meet their daily needs. Supplementing with cyanocobalamin, a synthetic form of vitamin B12, is only beneficial when there is a deficiency of vitamin B12 (Jelkmann, 2012). However, despite its common use, supplemental cyanocobalamin is typically unnecessary. Vitamin-mineral supplements should only be utilized when a horse's diet has a known deficiency in a specific vitamin or mineral after consideration of the vitamin and mineral composition of the compound feed and the forage. It is important to assess the nutritional composition of the horse's feed before introducing supplements to prevent imbalances or potential toxicity, as toxicity has been observed with minerals like selenium or iodine and fat-soluble vitamins A and D. Feeding compound feeds at lower-than-recommended rates may lead to a need for supplementary minerals and vitamins.

Amino acid supplements: The synthesis of body proteins relies on a specific ratio of amino acids. Although the true dietary requirement is for amino acids rather than protein itself, the individual amino acid requirements for horses are not well defined at present. Currently, only lysine, widely recognized as the first limiting amino acid in horses, has a recommended value published in the NRC guidelines. A limiting amino acid is an essential amino acid provided in the lowest amount relative to its requirement, thereby impeding protein synthesis. Even if the other amino acids are adequately or abundantly supplied, protein synthesis cannot proceed if a limiting amino acid is not present. In a typical equine diet composed of grasses and cereal grains, lysine and threonine have been identified as the most limiting amino acids, and they are often supplemented in horse feeds to supply requirements for growth and enhance body protein synthesis (Graham et al., 1994; Ott et al., 1981). Supplementing growing horses with additional lysine has been shown to increase the growth rate in lysine-deficient diets (Ott et al., 1981), while threonine supplementation has resulted in greater girth gain (Graham et al., 1994). Supplementation of lysine and threonine together in mature horses has been found to improve muscle mass scores and reduce body condition scores without affecting BW (Graham-Thiers & Kronfeld, 2005). For many sedentary horses, a diet consisting of high-quality forage can meet their overall protein requirements. However, if there is a need or desire for muscle development, a higher-quality protein source can be a valuable addition to their diet. Supplementing these specific amino acids can be considered to provide additional amino acids if the horse's current diet does not meet the dietary requirements. Consumption of a higher-quality protein source, such as soy-based protein supplements, can provide a stronger anabolic signal to activate muscle protein synthesis pathways than lower-quality forage-based protein sources.

Specialized dietary supplements

A specialized dietary supplement is a substance that is orally consumed by horses, either mixed with feed or offered separately, to provide specific benefits to the horses beyond providing essential nutrients or meeting normal nutritional needs. These substances do not fall under the category of legally defined drugs. This definition encompasses various nutraceuticals and other nutrients that are often recommended for their perceived significant effects on horses' health, performance, and behavior (Harris & Dunnett, 2018). The most common ones are:

Probiotics and prebiotics: Probiotics are naturally present in various food sources. Yogurt, in particular, contains several common strains of probiotic bacteria, and some products are fortified with additional cultures. Other fermented foods like sauerkraut and kimchi are also rich in probiotics. For horses, probiotics are available as powdered, pelleted, or liquid feed supplements.

Probiotics are believed to support a horse's health in several ways:

- Stimulation of the immune system: Probiotics support the immune response by activating intracellular signaling pathways within the intestinal epithelial cells.
- Production of antimicrobial substances: Probiotics secrete antimicrobial metabolites, such as acetic acid and lactic acid, which can kill pathogens. These organic acids exhibit strong inhibitory effects on gram-negative bacteria.
- Reduction of "bad" bacteria through competitive exclusion: Beneficial probiotic strains compete with potentially harmful bacteria for space on the intestinal mucous membrane, preventing pathogens from adhering or entering epithelial cells. Probiotics block receptors on surface cells and increase the production of mucin, a component of mucus that helps prevent pathogen attachment.
- Inhibition or inactivation of bacterial toxins: Probiotics can hinder gene expression in bacteria that produce or release toxins in the gut.

Considering these potential beneficial actions, probiotics are often administered to horses to support overall health during periods of stress or recovery from illness. Each probiotic product has a specific formulation of microorganisms, which should be listed on the product label. The most common probiotic groups include *Lactobacillus*, *Bifidobacterium*, *Enterococcus*, and yeasts like *Saccharomyces*. Different types of probiotics may be labeled for specific effects, and many contain a combination of different bacterial strains to provide a range of benefits.

Fortunately, studies have shown that administering up to three times the manufacturer's recommended doses of probiotics to healthy horses had no adverse effects, making overdosing unlikely. However, it is important to note that commercial probiotics are not regulated, so buyers should exercise caution and be mindful of their choices. Several studies have found that most label claims for probiotics' contents are not met (Weese & Martin, 2011).

A recent review (Cooke et al., 2021) summarized the current evidence on the safety and efficacy of probiotic bacteria use in horses. No clear benefits were identified to support supplementing with probiotic bacteria to improve digestion, treat colic, or prevent salmonellosis. Conflicting results were seen with the management of scouring in neonatal foals. Exacerbation of pre-existing diarrhea and additional adverse events were reported after administration of high doses of novel probiotic bacterial species. Most bacterial species used in equine probiotics are commonly used for human consumption and indigenous to the human gastrointestinal microbiota, so selection of equine-specific bacteria may give better results. There is currently a lack of evidence to support the use of probiotic bacteria in the health maintenance and disease management of horses.

It's important not to confuse probiotics with prebiotics, as they serve different functions in the gastrointestinal tract. Prebiotics typically refer to complex carbohydrates that serve as metabolic fuel for microorganisms in the gut. They provide energy specifically to the beneficial bacteria in the gastrointestinal tract. In simpler terms, prebiotics can be seen as the "food" for the microbiota. However, strong evidence suggests that certain unprotected prebiotics, such as FOS (fructoligosaccharides) and inulin, do not fully survive the journey through the stomach and small intestine (Bachmann et al., 2019). Instead, they undergo fermentation and partial degradation in the stomach due to microbial fermentation and acid. This elevated fermentation in the stomach may potentially have a significant impact on stomach health.

Joint supplements: Given the prevalence of lameness and osteoarthritis as common equine ailments, it is unsurprising that joint supplementation is widely used among performance horse owners and trainers (Agar et al., 2016). Osteoarthritis is a disease characterized by structural and functional changes in synovial joints, resulting from an imbalance between the synthesis and degradation of essential substances in the joints. Commercial joint supplements for horses typically contain a combination of nutrients, nutrient derivatives, and herbs. Among the numerous products marketed as joint supplements, the most common "active ingredients" found in them are glucosamine and chondroitin sulfate. The body naturally synthesizes both substances, and they are present in high quantities in joint cartilage, synovial fluid, and vertebral discs. Therefore, the necessity for supplementation with these substances is a subject of controversy. They have been extensively studied for their potential in preventing and treating osteoarthritis, but their effectiveness remains debatable. Although there is no official standard recommended dosage of glucosamine for horses, some studies have suggested a dosage of around 10,000 mg/day for a mature horse (Laverty et al., 2005). Glucosamine is available in two distinct forms: HCL (hydrochloride) and sulfate. However, it should be noted that many of the supplements available on the market do not provide the required dosage levels of glucosamine and chondroitin for horses.

In a recent study, horses were given a supplement containing chondroitin sulfate, glucosamine, vitamin C, methyl sulphonyl methane (MSM), DHA, EPA, or a placebo in their feed for 21 days in a triple-blind crossover design. The study found that oral administration of this supplement was associated with reduced lameness, improved ridden/groundwork scores, and enhanced ease of movement in the field (Murray et al., 2013).

Hoof supplements: Biotin, a water-soluble B vitamin, is the primary ingredient found in equine hoof supplements. Nutrients such as biotin, copper (Cu), zinc (Zn), manganese (Mn), and methionine have been previously shown to improve the quality and growth rates of horse hoof horn, leading to the production of healthier hoof walls (Ott & Johnson, 2001). Biotin plays a crucial role in the production of keratin, which is an intracellular protein that provides mechanical resilience and waterproofing capacity to epithelial cells. Horses have a low daily biotin requirement, but much higher amounts are required to stimulate rapid hoof growth, such as 20 mg/600 kg (Reilly et al., 1998). Similarly, copper, zinc, and manganese are important for keratinization and cell-to-cell adhesion processes (Tomlinson et al., 2004). A deficiency in these nutrients and protein/amino acids can negatively impact hoof growth and quality. Supplementation with organic trace minerals led to greater hoof growth than seen with similar levels for inorganic minerals, although there was no effect on hoof strength (Ott & Johnson, 2001).

A recent study (Suagee-Bedore et al., 2022) investigated the effects of flaxseed, a source of ALA, trace minerals, and biotin, on hoof growth. The study found that supplementing with flaxseed, copper, zinc, manganese, and biotin for 32 weeks provided additional nutrients in the diet and enhanced hoof growth in the front hooves. Unpublished data (Huntington pers comm) using a biotin, organic zinc, methionine, and lecithin supplement for 200 days found a 17% increase in hoof growth in six horses compared to control horses. Marked differences were seen in winter and summer. The fatty acid profile of hoof tissue is similar to that of skin, containing fatty acids that contribute to its waterproofing function. Hoof tissue, being an epithelial tissue, is rich in saturated fats like stearic acid (18:0) and palmitic acid (16:0), as well as omega-9 fatty acid oleic acid (18:1 n9) and omega-6 fatty acid linoleic acid (18:2 n6), all of which contribute to its waterproofing capacity (Elias, 1981). It is still unknown whether it is possible to alter the fatty acid profile of hoof tissue or the effect of this modification.

Ulcer supplements: Multiple products are available for treating and preventing of equine gastric ulcers. Squamous ulcers, which are part of the equine gastric ulcer syndrome, are common, with a prevalence ranging from 60% to 90% (Vatistas et al., 1999), while increasing use of endoscopy is detecting more glandular ulcer disease. In recent years, there has been a growing interest in the use of feed supplements to manage gastric ulcers in horses, and numerous commercial products are now available. Here are some significant findings from research on ulcer treatment and prevention supplements:

- A proton pump inhibitor has demonstrated effectiveness in treating and preventing gastric ulcers (Andrews et al., 1999).
- Porcine hydrolyzed collagen, when fed as a supplement to horses along with omeprazole, has shown enhanced effects on increasing gastric juice pH, inhibiting gastrin secretion after feeding, and reducing the incidence of squamous ulcers in stall-confined horses undergoing intermittent feeding over a long-term period (56 days) (Camacho-Luna et al., 2022).
- Pectin, a soluble complex polysaccharide derived from fruits and vegetables, and lecithin, a phospholipid derived from soybeans with surfactant properties, form a hydrophobic barrier on the gastric mucosal membranes when combined. This combination, found in supplements, has been shown to decrease the severity of squamous gastric ulcers compared to untreated control horses. Previous studies have also reported reduced squamous gastric ulcer severity after 10 to 35 days of treatment with pectin and lecithin-containing supplements (Woodward et al., 2014).
- A marine-derived calcium supplement has buffering effects on the equine gastric environment. It has been observed that these buffering effects are significant within 2 hours of consumption and can persist for up to 4 hours in some horses (Jacobs et al., 2020).
- Feeding a proprietary mineral complex containing calcified *Lithothamnion corallioides* and *Phymatolithon calcareum*, types of red algae, has been shown to reduce the prevalence of gastric ulcers in stressed horses. In a field trial involving mature draft geldings, horses that received the proprietary mineral complex had a lower number of squamous ulcers and a trend for fewer glandular ulcers compared to horses without added mineral supplementation (Gordon et al., 2017).
- Supplementation with a blend of fish/safflower oil for 84 days significantly reduced the severity of squamous ulceration in horses in race training. However, this effect was not seen with a flax/corn oil blend supplying the same levels of omega-3 and omega-6 fatty acids (Pagan et al., 2022).

Calmers for horses: The proper functioning of the nervous system relies on various vitamins and minerals, such as B vitamins, calcium, and magnesium. Deficiencies in these nutrients can lead to behavioral problems in horses. Supplementation with vitamin B1 and magnesium has shown reduced anxiety and stress markers (Pearson & MacNicol, 2017), and supplemental magnesium has been shown to reduce reaction speed (Dodd et al., 2015). Tryptophan is another commonly used ingredient in equine calming supplements (Grimmett & Sillence, 2005). Tryptophan serves as a precursor to serotonin, a neurotransmitter associated with feelings of relaxation and well-being, and low serotonin levels have been linked to anxiety and nervousness. However, some research has shown tryptophan can be excitatory. As a result, many commercial calming supplements combine these elements to promote a calming effect in horses.

Electrolytes and rehydration for horses: Electrolytes are widely used in performance horses (Agar et al., 2016; Burk & Williams, 2008). They are mineral salts that dissolve in the bloodstream and various bodily fluids, and they are naturally lost through urine, saliva, bile, mucus, intestinal tract secretions, and sweat on a daily basis.

There are three categories of electrolytes commonly recognized:

- Major electrolytes, which include sodium, potassium, and chloride. Sodium chloride is commonly referred to as salt and potassium chloride is lite salt. Iodized salt also contains small amounts of iodine.
- Minor electrolytes, which consist of calcium and magnesium.
- Trace electrolytes, such as zinc, copper, and iron (Bishop, 2005).

Horses that engage in activities causing significant sweating do not necessarily require electrolyte supplementation as they may be getting adequate intakes of electrolytes from salt, forage, and feed. However, horses that have undergone intense or prolonged exercise, have been exposed to hot or humid weather, or have traveled long distances may need some form of electrolyte supplementation to restore their electrolyte levels to an adequate balance. It is important to note that electrolytes cannot be preloaded in horses, so electrolyte supplements are typically given during and after exercise. Regardless of the weather or exercise conditions, horses should have daily access to salt blocks or have loose salt added to their feed.

Sodium (Na), chloride (Cl), and potassium (K) are vital components of a horse's diet. Potassium deficiency is uncommon in horses due to high levels of this essential mineral in hay, pasture, and various high-fiber ingredients. Offering horses daily access to salt as a block or rock salt or regularly providing salt often guarantees that their essential sodium requirements for hydration are met. Sodium chloride is the primary source of sodium, and it is available in various forms, such as iodized salt, sea salt, Himalayan salt, and more. It is advisable always to have salt accessible to horses, and horses do have some nutritional wisdom regarding free-choice salt intake. An average 500-kg horse requires 10 grams of sodium and 40 grams of chloride on a cool day doing no work (NRC), 2007). Feeding 30 grams of salt a day will provide 11.7 grams of sodium, enough to meet the maintenance needs of a 500-kg horse. Within the brain, there are detectors responsible for regulating the concentration of sodium in the blood. Should sodium levels in circulation rise, a sensation of thirst is initiated, prompting the intake of water. Water constitutes slightly more than 60% of a horse's BW and plays a critical role in a multitude of physiological processes. Ensuring an appropriate sodium level is crucial not only for neuromuscular functions but also for the overall state of hydration.

Immune support supplements: Antioxidants, omega-3 oils, and certain herbal-based supplements are commonly used to support the immune system in horses.

- Omega-3 fatty acids are well-known for their immune-boosting properties (Vineyard et al., 2010). Since horses cannot synthesize these fatty acids, they must be included in their diet.
- Some herbal-based supplements have been shown to stimulate inflammatory immune responses, with the blue-green algae *Spirulina platensis* specifically enhancing the production of immunoglobulin G antibodies (Nawrocka et al., 2017). Brewer's yeast beta-glucan supplements have been found to significantly stimulate non-specific defense mechanisms and enhance both non-specific and specific immune responses after vaccination in horses with some vaccines (Rakebrandt et al., 2023).
- Antioxidants are used widely as immune supporters. They are administered to horses to counteract the harmful effects of oxidative stress caused by pathological conditions or physical exercise. Oxidative stress refers to the excessive generation of free radicals, which can damage the horse's health. Free radicals disrupt the balance of stable molecules and contribute to inflammation and tissue damage. Adding vitamins E, C, and β-carotene to the horses' diets in stressful conditions can reduce the production of free radicals associated with oxidative stress (Garcia et al., 2022). Older horses with reduced immune function are also candidates for supplementation. Common antioxidant supplements include vitamin E, vitamin C, and selenium, as these nutrients are often deficient in horse diets. Natural vitamin E offers superior bioavailability compared to synthetic vitamin E, and certain nano-dispersed liquid forms have been shown to be capable of rapidly increasing serum levels of this vitamin (Huntington et al., 2013). The horse makes vitamin C in the liver, but additional amounts may be indicated in certain conditions. The form (injectable or oral) and the amount required daily of supplementary vitamin C are uncertain.

Performance or ergogenic supplements: Although there are claims that performance supplements can enhance performance or improve health, there is a lack of evidence-based studies to support these claims. Therefore, performance supplements in this context refer to those designed to provide extra energy, increase stamina, and improve aerobic capabilities in horses. Examples of such supplements include creatine, maltodextrin, and fats and oils.

- Creatine is involved in replenishing ATP (adenosine triphosphate), which plays a crucial role in providing energy for muscle contraction. However, the effects of dietary creatine supplementation on performance in horses are controversial. For instance, a study by Schuback et al. (2000) found no enhancement in the performance of horses during maximal treadmill exercise when supplemented with creatine. Some studies have also investigated the impact of oral creatine supplementation on muscular creatine phosphate reserves in horses, but have not observed any significant effects. This lack of effect has been attributed to the low oral bioavailability of creatine in horses (Schubak et al., 2000).
- Maltodextrin is believed to enhance a horse's performance by providing additional energy, which can delay the onset of fatigue (Jose-Cunilleras et al., 2002). However, there is a lack of clinical studies to support these theories.
- Oils are often included in the horses' diets of to increase energy content while potentially enhancing their athletic capacity (Geor, 2006). However, the specific effects of oils on performance have not been extensively studied in clinical research. Work at the University of Kentucky (O'Connor et al., 2004) found that fish oil supplementation led to lower heart rates during strenuous exercise. Oil source may have an impact as Kennedy et al. (1999) replaced corn oil iso-energetically with rice bran in the diet of horses performing strenuous exercise and found that horses had significantly lower heart rates during a standardized exercise test (SET) and lower plasma lactate at the end of the SET.

Herbal supplements: Herbal supplements for horses have become increasingly popular and mainstream over the past four decades, as is the case with their use among humans. While most herbs have cumulative and slow-acting effects on horses, it is crucial to acknowledge that herbal products can still lead to imbalances or overdoses, and some contain drugs that can contravene rules about the detection of prohibited substances. Merely labeling a product as "herbal" or "natural" does not guarantee its safety. It is essential to carefully read the labels of herbal products, know what ingredients are in the supplement, and follow the dosage instructions just as diligently as one would for any medication, although most dosage instructions are not based on controlled research into dose responses or safety.

Following is a list of the most commonly utilized herbal supplements in equine nutrition (Elghandour et al., 2018).

- **Devil's claw:** Devil's claw is rich in a compound called harpagoside, which possesses anti-inflammatory properties. In equine supplements, devil's claw is commonly included in joint-support products. While research on its efficacy is still pending, a pharmacokinetic study conducted in 2018 showed that the active ingredient entered the blood of horses within 30 minutes of administration, with no clinically detectable adverse side effects (Torfs et al., 2008). However, caution should be exercised as devil's claw is a bitter herb that can increase gastric secretions, making it potentially unsuitable for horses with a history of gastric ulcers.
- **Echinacea:** Echinacea contains active components such as caffeic acid derivatives, polysaccharides, and alkamides. A Canadian study conducted in 2002 demonstrated that echinacea extract increased red blood cell and hemoglobin levels in healthy horses, while also stimulating white blood cell function (O'Neill et al., 2002). The researchers speculated that this could potentially enhance athletic performance. Currently, no specific safety or dosing information regarding echinacea is available for horses.
- **Evening primrose oil:** Evening primrose oil is rich in unsaturated fatty acids, including linoleic, gamma-linoleic, palmitic, and oleic acids, which are considered beneficial dietary fats. Anecdotal reports from horse owners suggest that primrose oil can help alleviate sweet itch in horses, but there is a lack of scientific studies confirming these observations. Currently, no specific dosing guidelines regarding the use of primrose oil have been established for horses.
- **Garlic:** Garlic is widely used in the horse industry. It is commonly included in products designed to repel pests such as flies, midges, mosquitoes, and ticks. Some horse owners also give garlic to horses with chronic respiratory conditions, believing it to have natural antibiotic properties. Feeding garlic to horses in large amounts can be harmful and lead to toxicity and Heinz body anemia, a condition caused by oxidative damage to red blood cells. Additionally, while some people claim that garlic acts as a "natural dewormer," no scientific evidence supports its antiparasitic properties. Relying on garlic instead of proven anthelmintic products puts horses at risk of internal parasite infestation.
- **Ginseng:** Ginseng products are marketed as stress reducers and performance enhancers. However, there is a scarcity of research conducted specifically on horses. One study conducted at the Equine Research Centre at the University of Guelph in Canada in 2007 examined the effects of low-dose dietary ginseng supplementation in healthy horses. The results showed that horses given this supplementation had increased antibody levels after vaccination against equine herpesvirus,

indicating that the herb might be a beneficial addition to vaccination protocols (Pearson et al., 2007). Currently, there are no recommended dosages or comprehensive studies on potential side effects in horses.

- **Ginger:** The active components found in ginger are known as gingerols and shogaols. A study conducted at Rutgers University in 2009 revealed that ginger extract could reduce the recovery time from peak fatigue to a post-exercise plateau in horses, which could benefit horses involved in physically demanding activities like racing or show jumping (Liburt et al., 2009). However, there is a lack of studies providing safe or recommended dosages. Additionally, ginger's caustic properties suggest that feeding it to horses with a history of gastric ulcers may not be advisable.
- **Rose hips:** Some "natural" rose hip powders are actually fortified with vitamin C and can be effective as an antioxidant agent in horses. Horses typically produce sufficient amounts of vitamin C in their liver and do not require supplementation. Nevertheless, some individuals believe that supplementing vitamin C may be beneficial for horses. A study conducted in Denmark in 2012 found evidence of increased antioxidant activity in harness racehorses that regularly received supplements containing rose hips (Winther et al., 2012).
- **Valerian:** In the equine industry, valerian root extract is marketed as a "calming" supplement aimed at alleviating nervousness, stress, and fear in horses without impacting their performance. However, there is a lack of scientific evidence to support these claims. Valerian is prohibited by many equestrian organizations, including the Fédération Equestre Internationale (FEI), and its use is not recommended.
- **Yucca:** Yucca extracts are believed to possess anti-inflammatory, antiarthritic, antioxidant, and antispasmodic effects. However, there is no reliable data confirming these claims in horses specifically. There are no established dosage guidelines for yucca in horses, and caution should be exercised when using yucca as a supplement.

Even if you don't consider yourself someone who uses herbal remedies for your horse, many owners have at least one plant-based product in the feed room that is used to promote your horse's health. However, it is vital to note that there is a lack of controlled scientific evidence about the efficacy, dosage, and safety of herbs, making the use of herbs a speculative practice.

2.6 Feeding frequency

Feed horses "little and often" to maintain a healthy gastrointestinal tract

Every horse has a fundamental and essential need for consistent intake of forage to maintain their behavioral, physical, and mental well-being. It is crucial to ensure that any disruption in feed intake does not exceed a period of 4 hours, as horses naturally prefer not to interrupt their feeding for longer periods (Baumgartner et al., 2020). Unfortunately, this fundamental need is often overlooked in practical settings.

Providing horses with more frequent meals can also aid in reducing or splitting their daily starch intake through their diet. It is advisable for horses to have a starch intake of <1.1 g/kg BW/meal, but it can be challenging to achieve, especially for high-performance horses that receive substantial grain feeds in their diet (Vervuert et al., 2009).

Research has shown that horses kept in individual housing with non-edible bedding, such as shavings, experienced an average nocturnal feed interruption of 9 hours, which can put their health at risk. Additionally, horses with non-edible bedding tended to consume their hay more quickly and with fewer breaks than those with edible bedding. When the horses' access to forage or bedding material like straw is limited, and their high-priority need for continuous feed intake is disregarded, they may exhibit accelerated consumption of forage and spend less time consuming their evening meal compared to horses with access to straw (Baumgartner et al., 2020).

It is crucial to address this situation to ensure the horses' well-being. Some alternatives to manage this issue include promoting the use of appropriate fiber sources and increasing the feeding time by adding sufficient chaff of the appropriate type and length or using double haynets with small access holes. However, it is important to note that unrestricted access to pasture can also pose risks, such as laminitis and obesity, if the energy intake exceeds the horses' requirements (Harris, 2007). Careful management is necessary to balance providing continuous access to forage and maintaining optimal health for the horses.

2.7 Feed storage guidelines

Most of the research on the hygienic quality of horse forage has primarily focused on the presence of mold, particularly when the hay is on the ground (Figure 2.11). Poor weather conditions during hay harvest, such as heavy rainfall and harvesting hay with high moisture content (over 20%), have been found to increase mold contamination during storage. Additionally, hay contaminated with soil has been shown to elevate mold levels and alter the diversity of fungi present (Séguin et al., 2010). Preservatives have been considered a viable option for improving hay quality during storage. Preservatives like propionic acid and lactic bacteria have traditionally been used in silage preservation, and some of these methods can be adapted for dry hay to inhibit mold growth (Reboux et al., 2002).

Implementing certain agricultural practices can also enhance hay quality. For example, practices such as eliminating molehills, baling at a moisture content of 850 g kg–1 FM (fresh matter), using barn drying, and applying propionic acid before baling, particularly when the hay still contains excess

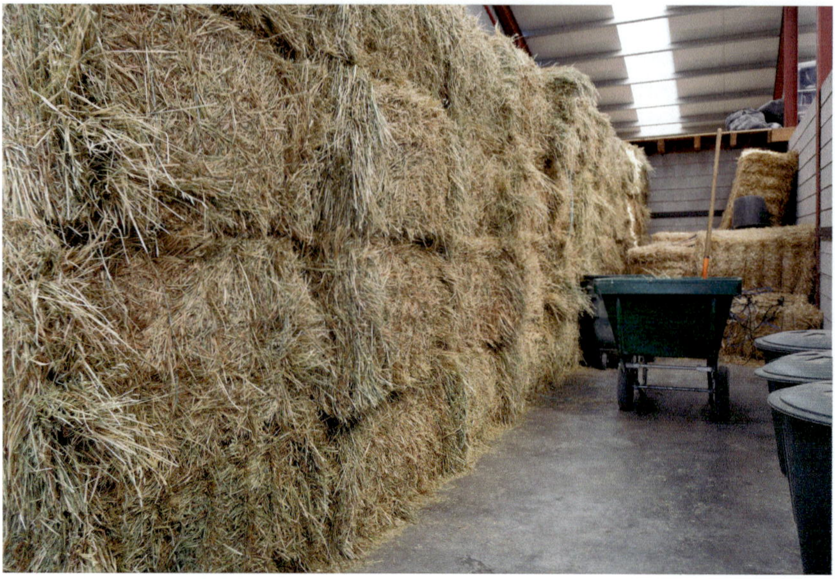

Figure 2.11 The forage storage.

moisture, have been shown to improve hay quality (Séguin et al., 2012). Additionally, tossing the hay after cutting will promote uniform drying before baling. Moreover, haylage, a form of preserved forage, appears to offer a favorable balance between nutritional value and health benefits.

The general feed storage guidelines:

- Store feed in a cool, dry, and well-ventilated area: High temperatures and humidity can accelerate feed deterioration and increase the risk of mold and bacterial growth. It is important to keep feed in a dry environment to maintain its quality and prevent spoilage. If feed gets wet, it is more prone to mold, and nutrients can be washed out of wet hay.
- Protect feed from pests: Store feed in tightly sealed containers or bins to prevent pests such as rodents and insects from accessing and contaminating the feed. Regularly inspect storage areas for signs of pest activity and take necessary measures to eliminate them.
- Use a first-in, first-out (FIFO) system: Practice proper stock rotation by using older feed first and placing newly purchased feed behind it. This helps to prevent feed from sitting in storage for extended periods, reducing the risk of spoilage and maintaining freshness.
- Avoid direct sunlight: Exposure to sunlight can cause feed to deteriorate and lose nutritional value. Store feed in a location shielded from direct sunlight or use opaque containers that block light.

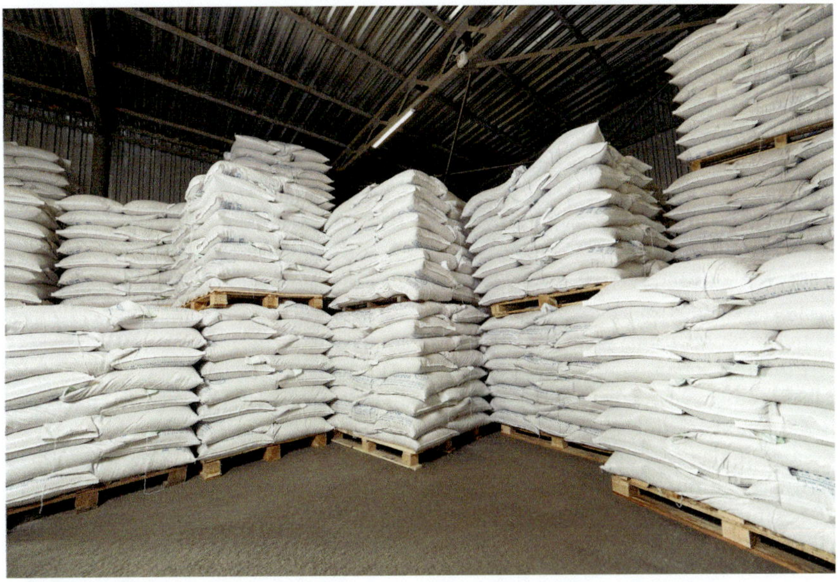

Figure 2.12 The feed storage.

- Keep feed off the ground: Elevate feed off the floor to prevent contact with moisture and potential contaminants. Use pallets or shelving to raise bags or containers of feed and provide proper airflow underneath. Hay is often stored on the ground, but there are some advantages to storing it off the ground on pallets (Figure 2.12).
- Check for signs of spoilage: Regularly inspect feed for mold, unusual odors, or pests. Discard any feed that appears moldy, has a foul smell, or shows signs of pest infestation.
- Follow the manufacturer's instructions: Read and follow the storage recommendations provided by the feed manufacturer. Different types of feed may have specific storage requirements, so it is important to adhere to the manufacturer's guidelines for optimal storage conditions.
- Ensure silage and haylage wraps are not damaged, as entry of air will result in mold.

By following these feed storage guidelines, you can help ensure the quality and safety of your horse's feed, promoting their health and well-being.

References

AAFCO (Association of American Feed Control Officials, Inc.). (2005). *Official Publication.*

Agar, C., Gemmill, R., Hollands, T., & Freeman, S. L. (2016). The use of nutritional supplements in dressage and eventing horses. *Veterinary Record Open*, *3*(1). https://doi.org/10.1136/vetreco-2015-000154

Andrews, F. M., Sifferman, R. L., Bernard, W., Hughes, F. E., Holste, J. E., Daurio, C. P., Alva, R., & Cox, J. L. (1999). Efficacy of omeprazole paste in the treatment and prevention of gastric ulcers in horses. *Equine Veterinary Journal*, *31*(S29), 81–86. https://doi.org/10.1111/j.2042-3306.1999.tb05176.x

Bachmann, M., Glatter, M., Bochnia, M., Greef, J. M., Breves, G., & Zeyner, A. (2019). Estimating compartmental and total tract apparent digestibility in horses using internal and external markers. *Livestock Science*, *223*, 16–23. https://doi.org/10.1016/j.livsci.2019.02.015

Baise, E., Habyarimana, J. A., Amory, H., Boemer, F., Douny, C., Gustin, P., Marcillaud-Pitel, C., Patarin, F., Weber, M., & Votion, D.-M. (2016). Samaras and seedlings of *Acer pseudoplatanus* are potential sources of hypoglycin A intoxication in atypical myopathy without necessarily inducing clinical signs. *Equine Veterinary Journal*, *48*(4), 414–417. https://doi.org/10.1111/evj.12499

Baumgartner, M., Boisson, T., Erhard, M. H., & Zeitler-Feicht, M. H. (2020). Common feeding practices pose a risk to the welfare of horses when kept on non-edible bedding. *Animals*, *10*(3), 411. https://doi.org/10.3390/ani10030411

Berny, P., Caloni, F., Croubels, S., Sachana, M., Vandenbroucke, V., Davanzo, F., & Guitart, R. (2010). Animal poisoning in Europe. Part 2: Companion animals. *The Veterinary Journal*, *183*(3), 255–259. https://doi.org/10.1016/j.tvjl.2009.03.034

Bishop, R. (2005). *The horse nutrition bible: The comprehensive guide to the correct feeding of your horse*. David & Charles.

Bochnia, M., Pietsch, C., Wensch-Dorendorf, M., Greef, M., & Zeyner, A. (2021). Effect of hay soaking duration on metabolizable energy, total and prececal digestible crude protein and amino acids, non-starch carbohydrates, macronutrients and trace elements. *Journal of Equine Veterinary Science*, *101*, 103452. https://doi.org/10.1016/j.jevs.2021.103452

Bott, R. C., Greene, E. A., Koch, K., Martinson, K. L., Siciliano, P. D., Williams, C., Trottier, N. L., Burk, A., & Swinker, A. (2013). Production and environmental implications of equine grazing. *Journal of Equine Veterinary Science*, *33*(12), 1031–1043. https://doi.org/10.1016/j.jevs.2013.05.004

Brooks, S. P. J., & Lampi, B. J. (2001). Problems associated with measuring phytate in infant cereals. *Journal of Agricultural and Food Chemistry*, *49*(2), 564–569. https://doi.org/10.1021/jf000715l

Burk, A. O., & Williams, C. A. (2008). Feeding management practices and supplement use in top-level event horses. *Comparative Exercise Physiology*, *5*(2), 85. https://doi.org/10.1017/S1478061508062786

Camacho-Luna, P., Andrews, F. M., Keowen, M. L., Garza, F., Liu, C. C., Lamp, B., & Olijve, J. (2022). The effect of porcine hydrolysed collagen on gastric ulcer scores, gastric juice pH, gastrin and amino acid concentrations in horses. *Equine Veterinary Education*, *34*(5), 248–257. https://doi.org/10.1111/eve.13409

Ceulemans, T., Merckx, R., Hens, M., & Honnay, O. (2011). A trait-based analysis of the role of phosphorus vs. nitrogen enrichment in plant species loss across North-west European grasslands. *Journal of Applied Ecology*, *48*(5), 1155–1163. https://doi.org/10.1111/j.1365-2664.2011.02023.x

Chatterton, N. J., Watts, K. A., Jensen, K. B., Harrison, P. A., & Horton, W. H. (2006). Nonstructural carbohydrates in oat forage. *The Journal of Nutrition*, *136*(7), 2111S–2113S. https://doi.org/10.1093/jn/136.7.2111S

Cooke, C. G., Gibb, Z., & Harnett, J. E. (2021). The safety, tolerability and efficacy of probiotic bacteria for equine use. *Journal of Equine Veterinary Science*, *99*, 103407. https://doi.org/10.1016/j.jevs.2021.103407

Coverdale, J. A., Moore, J. A., Tyler, H. D., & Miller-Auwerda, P. A. (2004). Soybean hulls as an alternative feed for horses. *Journal of Animal Science*, *82*(6), 1663–1668. https://doi.org/10.2527/2004.8261663x

Crandell, K. G., Pagan, J. D., Harris, P., & Duren, S. E. (1999). A comparison of grain, oil and beet pulp as energy sources for the exercised horse. *Equine Veterinary Journal*, *31*(S30), 485–489. https://doi.org/10.1111/j.2042-3306.1999.tb05270.x

Dänicke, S., Saltzmann, J., Liermann, W., Glatter, M., Hüther, L., Kersten, S., Zeyner, A., Feige, K., & Warnken, T. (2021). Evaluation of inner exposure of horses to Zearalenone (ZEN), Deoxynivalenol (DON) and their metabolites in relation to colic and health-related clinical-chemical traits. *Toxins (Basel)*, *13*(8), 588. https://doi.org/10.3390/toxins13080588

Daniel, A. D., McIntosh, B. J., Plunk, J. D., Webb, M., McIntosh, D., & Parks, A. G. (2015). 7 Effects of rotational grazing on water-soluble carbohydrate and energy content of horse pastures. *Journal of Equine Veterinary Science*, *35*(5), 385–386. https://doi.org/10.1016/j.jevs.2015.03.014

Desjardins, A. E., Hohn, T. M., & McCormick, S. P. (1993). Trichothecene biosynthesis in Fusarium species: Chemistry, genetics, and significance. *Microbiological Reviews*, *57*(3), 595–604. https://doi.org/10.1128/mr.57.3.595-604.1993

Dodd, J. A., Doran, G., Harris, P., & Noble, G. K. (2015). 41 Magnesium aspartate supplementation and reaction speed response in horses. *Journal of Equine Veterinary Science*, *35*(5), 401–402. https://doi.org/10.1016/j.jevs.2015.03.051

Edouard, N., Fleurance, G., Martin-Rosset, W., Duncan, P., Dulphy, J. P., Grange, S., Baumont, R., Dubroeucq, H., Pérez-Barbería, F. J., & Gordon, I. J. (2008). Voluntary intake and digestibility in horses: Effect of forage quality with emphasis on individual variability. *Animal*, *2*(10), 1526–1533. https://doi.org/10.1017/S1751731108002760

European Food Safety Authority. (2004a). Opinion of the scientific panel on contaminants in the food chain on a request from the commission related to deoxynivalenol (DON) as undesirable substance in animal feed. *European Food Safety Authority Journal*, 73, 1–42. http://www.efsa.europa.eu (accessed 15 October 2009)

European Food Safety Authority. (2004b). Opinion of the Scientific Panel on Contaminants in the Food Chain on a request from the Commission related to fumonisins as undesirable substances in animal feed. *European Food Safety Authority Journal*, 235, 1–32. https://doi.org/10.2903/j.efsa.2005.235

European Food Safety Authority. (2004c). Opinion of the scientific panel on contaminants in the food chain on a request from the commission related to ochratoxin A (OTA) as undesirable substance in animal feed. *European Food Safety Authority Journal*, *101*, 1–36. http://www.efsa.europa.eu (accessed 15 October 2009)

Elghandour, M. M. M. Y., Kanth Reddy, P. R., Salem, A. Z. M., Ranga Reddy, P. P., Hyder, I., Barbabosa-Pliego, A., & Yasaswini, D. (2018). Plant bioactives and extracts as feed additives in horse nutrition. *Journal of Equine Veterinary Science*, *69*, 66–77. https://doi.org/10.1016/j.jevs.2018.06.004

Elias, P. M. (1981). Epidermal lipids, membranes, and keratinization. *International Journal of Dermatology*, *20*(1), 1–19. https://doi.org/10.1111/j.1365-4362.1981.tb05278.x

Evans, J. L. (1995). Forages for horses. In R. F. Barnes, D. A. Miller, & C. J. Nelson (Eds.), *Forages: The science of grassland agriculture* (5th ed., pp. 301–311). Iowa State University Press.

Evans, T. J. (2002). Endocrine alterations associated with ergopeptine alkaloid exposure during equine pregnancy. *Veterinary Clinics of North America: Equine Practice*, *18*(2), 371–378. https://doi.org/10.1016/S0749-0739(02)00019-6

Fink-Gremmels, J. (2008). The impact of mycotoxins in animal feeds. In *Mycotoxins: Detection methods, management, public health and agricultural trade* (pp. 155–167). CABI. https://doi.org/10.1079/9781845930820.0155

Garcia, E. I. C., Elghandour, M. M. M. Y., Khusro, A., Alcala-Canto, Y., Tirado-González, D. N., Barbabosa-Pliego, A., & Salem, A. Z. M. (2022). Dietary supplements of vitamins E, C, and β-Carotene to reduce oxidative stress in horses: An overview. *Journal of Equine Veterinary Science*, *110*, 103863. https://doi.org/10.1016/j.jevs.2022.103863

Geor, R., Harris, P., & Coenen, M. (2013). *Equine applied and clinical nutrition*. Elsevier Saunders.

Geor, R. J. (2006). The role of nutritional supplements and feeding strategies in equine athletic performance. *Equine and Comparative Exercise Physiology*, *3*(3), 109–119. https://doi.org/10.1017/ECP200690

Geor, R. J. (2010). Current concepts on the pathophysiology of pasture-associated laminitis. *Veterinary Clinics of North America: Equine Practice*, *26*(2), 265–276. https://doi.org/10.1016/j.cveq.2010.06.001

Gillman, J. H., Hegeman, A. D., & Sharp, R. G. (2014). Clarifying the role of maples in atypical myopathy. *Equine Veterinary Journal*, *46*, 135–136. doi: 10.1111/evj.12176.

Gimeno, A., & Quintavilla, J. A. (1983). Analytical and mycotoxicological study of a natural outbreak of zearalenone mycotoxicosis in horse. *Proceeding of International Symposium on Mycotoxins*, 387–392. Cairo, Egypt: National Research Centre.

Gordon, M. E., Vineyard, K. R., & Andrews, F. M. (2017). The effect of a natural-source mineral supplement on gastric juice pH in horses. *Journal of Equine Veterinary Science*, *52*, 58. https://doi.org/10.1016/j.jevs.2017.03.056

Graham, P. M., Ott, E. A., Brendemuhl, J. H., & TenBroeck, S. H. (1994). The effect of supplemental lysine and threonine on growth and development of yearling horses. *Journal of Animal Science*, *72*(2), 380–386. https://doi.org/10.2527/1994.722380x

Graham-Thiers, P. M., & Kronfeld, D. S. (2005). Amino acid supplementation improves muscle mass in aged and young horses. *Journal of Animal Science*, *83*(12), 2783–2788. https://doi.org/10.2527/2005.83122783x

Grimmett, A., & Sillence, M. N. (2005). Calmatives for the excitable horse: A review of L-tryptophan. *The Veterinary Journal*, *170*(1), 24–32. https://doi.org/10.1016/j.tvjl.2004.04.017

Hansen, D. K., Webb, G. W., & Webb, S. P. (1992). Digestibility of wheat straw or ammoniated wheat straw in equine diets. *Journal of Equine Veterinary Science*, *12*(4), 223–226. https://doi.org/10.1016/S0737-0806(06)81450-4

Harris, P., & Dunnett, C. (2018). Nutritional tips for veterinarians. *Equine Veterinary Education*, *30*(9), 486–496. https://doi.org/10.1111/eve.12657

Harris, P. A. (2007). How should we feed horses--and how many times a day? *Veterinary Journal (London, England : 1997)*, *173*(2), 252–253.

Harris, P. A., Ellis, A. D., Fradinho, M. J., Jansson, A., Julliand, V., Luthersson, N., Santos, A. S., & Vervuert, I. (2017). Review: Feeding conserved forage to horses: Recent advances and recommendations. *Animal*, *11*(6), 958–967. https://doi.org/10.1017/S1751731116002469

Henning, J., Lehmkuhler, J., Smith, R., Lacefield, G., Burris, R., Ditsch, D., & Coleman, B. (2000). Rotational grazing. *University of Kentucky Cooperative Extension Service ID-143*.

Hess, T. M., Rexford, J., Hansen, D. K., Ahrens, N. S., Harris, M., Engle, T., Ross, T., & Allen, K. G. (2013). Effects of Ω-3 (n-3) fatty acid supplementation on insulin sensitivity in horses. *Journal of Equine Veterinary Science*, *33*(6), 446–453. https://doi.org/10.1016/j.jevs.2012.07.007

Hoffman, C. J., Costa, L. R., & Freeman, L. M. (2009). Survey of feeding practices, supplement use, and knowledge of equine nutrition among a subpopulation of horse owners in New England. *Journal of Equine Veterinary Science*, *29*(10), 719–726. https://doi.org/10.1016/j.jevs.2009.08.005

Hoffman, R. M., Wilson, J. A., Kronfeld, D. S., Cooper, W. L., Lawrence, L. A., Sklan, D., & Harris, P. A. (2001). Hydrolyzable carbohydrates in pasture, hay, and horse feeds: Direct assay and seasonal variation. *Journal of Animal Science*, *79*(2), 500. https://doi.org/10.2527/2001.792500x

Holland, J. L., Kronfeld, D. S., Rich, G. A., Kline, K. A., Fontenot, J. P., Meacham, T. N., & Harris, P. A. (1998). Acceptance of fat and lecithin containing diets by horses. *Applied Animal Behaviour Science*, *56*(2–4), 91–96. https://doi.org/10.1016/S0168-1591(97)00101-9

Hongo, A., & Akimoto, M. (2003). The role of incisors in selective grazing by cattle and horses. *The Journal of Agricultural Science*, *140*(4), 469–477. https://doi.org/10.1017/S0021859603003083

Huntington, P. J., Pagan, J. D., Lawrence, T. L., & Lennox, M. A. (2010). Fish oil and corn oil supplementation affect red blood cell and serum EPA and DHA concentrations in thoroughbred horses. *Australian Equine Veterinarian*, *29*, 73.

Huntington, P. J., Pagan, J. D., Waldridge, B. M., Lange, J., & Brown-Douglas, C. G. (2013). Fish oil supplementation attenuates glucose intolerance caused by high dietary fat intake in aged thoroughbred geldings. *Australian Equine Veterinarian*, *32*(3), 44.

Hyslop, J. J., Jessop, N. S., Stefansdottir, G. J., & Cuddeford, D. (1997). Comparative degradation in situ of four concentrate feeds in the caecum of ponies and the lumen of steers. *Proceedings of the Fifteenth Equine Nutrition and Physiology Symposium*, 116–117.

Intemann, S., Reckels, B., Schubert, D., Wolf, P., Kamphues, J., & Visscher, C. (2022). The hygienic status of different forage types for horses—A retrospective study on influencing factors and associations with anamnestic reports. *Veterinary Sciences*, *9*(5), 226. https://doi.org/10.3390/vetsci9050226

Jacobs, R. D., Gordon, M. B. E., Vineyard, K. R., Keowen, M. L., Garza, F., & Andrews, F. M. (2020). The effect of a seaweed-derived calcium supplement on gastric juice pH in the horse. *Journal of Equine Veterinary Science*, *95*, 103265. https://doi.org/10.1016/j.jevs.2020.103265

Jansson, A., Harris, P., Davey, S. L., Luthersson, N., Ragnarsson, S., & Ringmark, S. (2021). Straw as an alternative to grass forage in horses—Effects on post-prandial metabolic profile, energy intake, behaviour and gastric ulceration. *Animals*, *11*(8), 2197. https://doi.org/10.3390/ani11082197

Jelkmann, W. (2012). The disparate roles of cobalt in erythropoiesis, and doping relevance. *Open Journal of Hematology*, *3*(1), 1. https://doi.org/10.13055/ojhmt_3_1_6.121211

Johnson, A. L., McAdams, S. C., & Whitlock, R. H. (2010). Type A botulism in horses in the United States: A review of the past ten years (1998–2008). *Journal of Veterinary Diagnostic Investigation: Official Publication of the American Association of Veterinary Laboratory Diagnosticians, Inc*, *22*(2), 165–173. https://doi.org/10.1177/104063871002200201

Jose-Cunilleras, E., Hinchcliff, K. W., Sams, R. A., Devor, S. T., & Linderman, J. K. (2002). Glycemic index of a meal fed before exercise alters substrate use and glucose flux in exercising horses. *Journal of Applied Physiology*, *92*(1), 117–128. https://doi.org/10.1152/jappl.2002.92.1.117

Julliand, V., De Fombelle, A., & Varloud, M. (2006). Starch digestion in horses: The impact of feed processing. *Livestock Science*, *100*(1), 44–52. https://doi.org/10.1016/j.livprodsci.2005.11.001

Kalantari, R. K., Rouzbehan, Y., Fazaeli, H., Direkvandi, E., & Salem, A. Z. M. (2021). The effect of three levels of concentrate and grain processing on feeding behavior, nutrient digestibility, blood metabolites and fecal pH of Turkmen horses. *Journal of Equine Veterinary Science*, *104*, 103690. https://doi.org/10.1016/j.jevs.2021.103690

Kamphues, J., Coenen, M., Kienzle, E., Pallauf, J., Simon, O., & Zentek, J. (2004). *Supplemente zu Vorlesungen und Übungen in der Tierernährung* (10th ed.). Schaper Philatelie Vlg, M&H.

Kellerman, T. S., Marasas, W. F., Thiel, P. G., Gelderblom, W. C., Cawood, M., & Coetzer, J. A. (1990). Leukoencephalomalacia in two horses induced by oral dosing of fumonisin B. *The Onderstepoort Journal of Veterinary Research*, *57*(4), 269–275.

Kennedy, M. A. P., Pagan, J. D., Hoekstra, K. E., Langfoss, E., & Heiderscheidt, K. (1999). An evaluation of corn oil, rice bran and refined dry fat as energy sources for exercised thoroughbreds. In: *Proc. 16th Equine Nutr. and Physiol. Soc. Symp.*, 130–113.

Kienzle, E., Pohlenz, J., & Radicke, S. (1997). Morphology of starch digestion in the horse. *Journal of Veterinary Medicine Series A*, *44*(1–10), 207–221. https://doi.org/10.1111/j.1439-0442.1997.tb01103.x

King, S. S., AbuGhazaleh, A. A., Webel, S. K., & Jones, K. L. (2008). Circulating fatty acid profiles in response to three levels of dietary omega-3 fatty acid supplementation in horses. *Journal of Animal Science*, *86*(5), 1114–1123. https://doi.org/10.2527/jas.2007-0682

Knudsen, K. E. B. (1997). Carbohydrate and lignin contents of plant materials used in animal feeding. *Animal Feed Science and Technology*, *67*(4), 319–338. https://doi.org/10.1016/S0377-8401(97)00009-6

Laverty, S., Sandy, J. D., Celeste, C., Vachon, P., Marier, J., & Plaas, A. H. K. (2005). Synovial fluid levels and serum pharmacokinetics in a large animal model following treatment with oral glucosamine at clinically relevant doses. *Arthritis & Rheumatism*, *52*(1), 181–191. https://doi.org/10.1002/art.20762

Liburt, N. R., McKeever, K. H., Streltsova, J. M., Franke, W. C., Gordon, M. E., Manso Filho, H. C., Horohov, D. W., Rosen, R. T., Ho, C. T., Singh, A. P., & Vorsa, N. (2009). Effects of ginger and cranberry extracts on the physiological response to exercise and markers of inflammation in horses. *Comparative Exercise Physiology*, 6(4), 157–169. https://doi.org/10.1017/S175525401000005X

Liesener, K., Curtui, V., Dietrich, R., Märtlbauer, E., & Usleber, E. (2010). Mycotoxins in horse feed. *Mycotoxin Research*, *26*(1), 23–30. https://doi.org/10.1007/s12550-009-0037-8

Longland, A. C., Barfoot, C., & Harris, P. A. (2011). The effect of wearing a grazing muzzle vs not wearing a grazing muzzle on pasture dry matter intake by ponies. *Journal of Equine Veterinary Science*, *31*(5–6), 282–283. https://doi.org/10.1016/j.jevs.2011.03.105

Longland, A. C., Ince, J., & Harris, P. A. (2011). Estimation of pasture intake by ponies from liveweight change during six weeks at pasture. *Journal of Equine Veterinary Science*, *31*(5–6), 275–276. https://doi.org/10.1016/j.jevs.2011.03.095

Lundqvist, H., & Elisabeth Müller, C. (2022). Feeding time in horses provided roughage in different combinations of haynets and on the stable floor. *Applied Animal Behaviour Science*, *253*, 105685. https://doi.org/10.1016/j.applanim.2022.105685

Martinson, K., Jung, H., Hathaway, M., & Sheaffer, C. (2012). The effect of soaking on carbohydrate removal and dry matter loss in Orchardgrass and Alfalfa Hays. *Journal of Equine Veterinary Science*, *32*(6), 332–338. https://doi.org/10.1016/j.jevs.2011.11.009

McNaughton, S. J. (1984). Grazing lawns: Animals in herds, plant form, and coevolution. *The American Naturalist*, *124*(6), 863–886. https://doi.org/10.1086/284321

Meerdink, G. L. (2002). Mycotoxins. *Clinical Techniques in Equine Practice*, *1*(2), 89–93. https://doi.org/10.1053/ctep.2002.34240

Meyer, H. (1992). *Pferdefütterung. 2. Auflage.* Verlag Paul Parey, Berlin und Hamburg

Meyer, H., Ahiswedeu, L., & Reinhardt, H. J. (1975). Studies on the duration of feeding, masticatory frequency and mincing of feed in horses. *DTW. Deutsche Tierarztliche Wochenschrift*, *82*(2), 54–58.

Meyer, H., Coenen, M., & Probst, D. (1986). Beiträge zur Verdauungsphysiologie des Pferdes. *Journal of Animal Physiology and Animal Nutrition*, *56*(1–5), 171–183. https://doi.org/10.1111/j.1439-0396.1986.tb00561.

Minervini, F., Giannoccaro, A., Nicassio, M., Panzarini, G., & Lacalandra, G. (2013). First evidence of placental transfer of Ochratoxin A in horses. *Toxins*, *5*(1), 84–92. https://doi.org/10.3390/toxins5010084

Molle, G., Cannas, A., & Gregorini, P. (2022). A review on the effects of part-time grazing herbaceous pastures on feeding behaviour and intake of cattle, sheep and horses. *Livestock Science*, *263*, 104982. https://doi.org/10.1016/j.livsci.2022.104982

Moore, J. E., Brant, M. H., Kunkle, W. E., & Hopkins, D. I. (1999). Effects of supplementation on voluntary forage intake, diet digestibility, and animal performance. *Journal of Animal Science*, *77*(suppl 2), 122. https://doi.org/10.2527/1999.77suppl_2122x

Moore-Colyer, M. J. S. (1996). Effects of soaking hay fodder for horses on dust and mineral content. *Animal Science*, *66*(03), 745–750. https://doi.org/10.1017/S1357729800009334

Mori, T. A., & Hodgson, J. M. (2013). Fatty acids: Health effects of Omega-6 polyunsaturated fatty acids. In *Encyclopedia of human nutrition* (pp. 209–214). Elsevier. https://doi.org/10.1016/B978-0-12-375083-9.00100-8

Morris, D. D., Henry, M. M., Moore, J. N., & Fischer, J. K. (1991). Effect of dietary alpha-linolenic acid on endotoxin-induced production of tumor necrosis factor by peritoneal macrophages in horses. *American Journal of Veterinary Research*, *52*(4), 528–532.

Muhonen, S., Sadet-Bourgeteau, S., & Julliand, V. (2021). Effects of differences in fibre composition and maturity of forage-based diets on the microbial ecosystem and its activity in equine caecum and colon digesta and faeces. *Animals*, *11*(8), 2337. https://doi.org/10.3390/ani11082337

Müller, C. E., Nostell, K., & Bröjer, J. (2015). Microbial counts in forages for horses—Effect of storage time and of water soaking before feeding. *Journal of Equine Veterinary Science*, *35*(7), 622–627. https://doi.org/10.1016/j.jevs.2015.06.005

Murray, R., Adams, V., Walker, V., Tranquille, C., Copeman, S., Spear, J., Frost, R., & Marlin, D. (2013). To determine the effect of an oral joint supplement on orthopaedic, physiotherapy and handler evaluation scores in horses. *Equine Veterinary Journal*, *45*(S44), 3–3. https://doi.org/10.1111/evj.12145_7

Myllykoski, J., Lindström, M., Keto-Timonen, R., Söderholm, H., Jakala, J., Kallio, H., Sukura, A., & Korkeala, H. (2009). Type C bovine botulism outbreak due to carcass contaminated non-acidified silage. *Epidemiology and Infection*, *137*(2), 284–293. https://doi.org/10.1017/S0950268808000939

National Research Council. (2007). *Nutrient requirements of horses* (6th ed.). National Academies Press. https://doi.org/10.17226/11653

Nawrocka, D., Kornicka, K., Śmieszek, A., & Marycz, K. (2017). Spirulina platensis improves mitochondrial function impaired by elevated oxidative stress in Adipose-Derived Mesenchymal Stromal Cells (ASCs) and Intestinal Epithelial Cells (IECs), and enhances insulin sensitivity in Equine Metabolic Syndrome (EMS) horses. *Marine Drugs*, *15*(8), 237. https://doi.org/10.3390/md15080237

Neuhaus, J., Schrödl, W., Shehata, A. A., & Krüger, M. (2015). Detection of Clostridium botulinum in liquid manure and biogas plant wastes. *Folia Microbiologica*, *60*(5), 451–456. https://doi.org/10.1007/s12223-015-0381-3

Nogradi, N., Couetil, L. L., Messick, J., Stochelski, M. A., & Burgess, J. R. (2015). Omega-3 fatty acid supplementation provides an additional benefit to a low-dust diet in the management of horses with chronic lower airway inflammatory disease. *Journal of Veterinary Internal Medicine*, *29*(1), 299–306. https://doi.org/10.1111/jvim.12488

O'Connor, C. I., Lawrence, L. M., Lawrence, A. C. St., Janicki, K. M., Warren, L. K., & Hayes, S. (2004). The effect of dietary fish oil supplementation on exercising horses. *Journal of Animal Science*, *82*(10), 2978–2984. https://doi.org/10.2527/2004.82102978x

O'Neill, W., McKee, S., & Clarke, A. F. (2002). Flaxseed (Linum usitatissimum) supplementation associated with reduced skin test lesional area in horses with Culicoides hypersensitivity. *Canadian Journal of Veterinary Research = Revue Canadienne de Recherche Veterinaire*, *66*(4), 272–277.

Ott, E. A., Asquith, R. L., & Feaster, J. P. (1981). Lysine supplementation of diets for yearling horses. *Journal of Animal Science*, *53*(6), 1496–1503. https://doi.org/10.2527/jas1982.5361496x

Ott, E. A., & Johnson, E. L. (2001). Effect of trace mineral proteinates on growth and skeletal and hoof development in yearling horses. *Journal of Equine Veterinary Science*, *21*(6), 287–291. https://doi.org/10.1016/S0737-0806(01)70059-7

Pagan, J. D., Hauss, A. A., Pagan, E. C., Simons, J. L., & Waldridge, B. M. (2022). Long-chain polyunsaturated fatty acid supplementation increases levels in red blood cells and reduces the prevalence and severity of squamous gastric ulcers in exercised Thoroughbreds. *Journal of the American Veterinary Medical Association*, *260*(S3), S121–S128. https://doi.org/10.2460/javma.22.06.0275

Pagan, J. D., & Mesquita, V. S. (2020). Feeding performance horses, in Proceedings. *Am Assoc Equine Pract*, *66*, 6674.

Pagan, J. D., Mesquita, V. S., Valberg, S. J., Waldridge, B., & Whitehouse, C. (2015). 58 Effect of non-structural carbohydrate intake on glycogen repletion following intense exercise. *Journal of Equine Veterinary Science*, *35*(5), 408–409. https://doi.org/10.1016/j.jevs.2015.03.068

Pearson, W., & MacNicol, J. (2017). Acute effects of a single-dose nutritional product on stress response and task completion in horses. *Journal of Equine Veterinary Science*, *51*, 86–91. https://doi.org/10.1016/j.jevs.2017.01.001

Pearson, W., Omar, S., & Clarke, A. F. (2007). Low-dose ginseng (Panax quinquefolium) modulates the course and magnitude of the antibody response to vaccination against equid herpesvirus I in horses. *Canadian Journal of Veterinary Research = Revue Canadienne de Recherche Veterinaire*, *71*(3), 213–217.

Pirie, R. S. (2014). Recurrent airway obstruction: A review. *Equine Veterinary Journal*, *46*(3), 276–288. https://doi.org/10.1111/evj.12204

Poole, D., & Erickson, H. (2016). Exercise-induced pulmonary hemorrhage: Where are we now? *Veterinary Medicine: Research and Reports*, *7*, 133–148. https://doi.org/10.2147/VMRR.S120421

Portier, K., de Moffarts, B., Fellman, N., Kirschvink, N., Motta, C., Letellier, C., Ruelland, A., Van Erck, E., Lekeux, P., & Coudert, J. (2006). The effects of dietary N-3 and antioxidant supplementation on erythrocyte membrane fatty acid composition and fluidity in exercising horses. *Equine Veterinary Journal*, *38*(S36), 279–284. https://doi.org/10.1111/j.2042-3306.2006.tb05553.x

Potter, G., Arnold, F., Householder, D., Hansen, D., & Bowen, K. (1992). Digestion of starch in the small or large intestine of the equine. *European Conference on Horse Nutrition*, 109–111.

Rakebrandt, M., Wróbel, M., & Siwicki, A. K. (2023). Influence of Brewer´s yeast beta-glucan supplementation on the non-specific defence mechanisms and specific immune response after Vaccination in Young Horses. *Proceedings of the Equine Health and Nutrition Congress Ghent*.

Reboux, G., Dalphin, J.-C., Polio, J.-C., Millon, L., Baverel, J., Martinez, J., Girard, L., & Piarroux, R. (2002). Influence of buffered propionic acid on the development of micro-organisms in hay. *Mycoses*, *45*(5–6), 184–187. https://doi.org/10.1046/j.1439-0507.2002.00754.x

Regulation. (2003). Regulation (EC) No 1831/2003 of the European Parliament and of the Council of 22 September 2003 on additives for use in animal nutrition. *OJ L 268, 18.10.2003*, 29–43.

Reilly, J. D., Cottrell, D. F., Martin, R. J., & Cuddeford, D. J. (1998). Effect of supplementary dietary biotin on hoof growth and hoof growth rate in ponies: A controlled trial. *Equine Veterinary Journal*, *30*(S26), 51–57. https://doi.org/10.1111/j.2042-3306.1998.tb05122.x

Richards, N., Hinch, G., & Rowe, J. (2006). The effect of current grain feeding practices on hindgut starch fermentation and acidosis in the Australian racing Thoroughbred. *Australian Veterinary Journal*, *84*(11), 402–407. https://doi.org/10.1111/j.1751-0813.2006.00059.x

Ropejko, K., & Twarużek, M. (2021). Zearalenone and its metabolites—General overview, occurrence, and toxicity. *Toxins*, *13*(1), 35. https://doi.org/10.3390/toxins13010035

Rotter, D., Prelusky, B., & Pestka, J. J. (1996). Toxicology of deoxynivalenol (vomitoxin). *Journal of Toxicology and Environmental Health*, *48*(1), 1–34. doi: 10.1080/009841096161447

Schmitz, A., Tonn, B., Schöppner, A.-K., & Isselstein, J. (2020). Using a citizen science approach with German horse owners to study the locomotion behaviour of horses on pasture. *Sustainability*, *12*(5), 1835. https://doi.org/10.3390/su12051835

Schuback, K., Essén-Gustavsson, B., & Persson, S. G. B. (2000). Effect of creatine supplementation on muscle metabolic response to a maximal treadmill exercise test in Standardbred horses. *Equine Veterinary Journal*, *32*(6), 533–540. https://doi.org/10.2746/042516400777584578

Séguin, V., Garon, D., Lemauviel-Lavenant, S., Lanier, C., Bouchart, V., Gallard, Y., Blanchet, B., Diquélou, S., Personeni, E., & Ourry, A. (2012). How to improve the hygienic quality of forages for horse feeding. *Journal of the Science of Food and Agriculture*, 92(4), 975–986. https://doi.org/10.1002/jsfa.4680

Séguin, V., Lemauviel-Lavenant, S., Garon, D., Bouchart, V., Gallard, Y., Blanchet, B., Diquelou, S., Personeni, E., Gauduchon, P., & Ourry, A. (2010). Effect of agricultural and environmental factors on the hay characteristics involved in equine respiratory disease. *Agriculture, Ecosystems & Environment*, *135*(3), 206–215. https://doi.org/10.1016/j.agee.2009.09.012

Siciliano, P. D., Gill, J. C., & Bowman, M. A. (2017). Effect of sward height on pasture nonstructural carbohydrate concentrations and blood glucose/insulin profiles in grazing Horses. *Journal of Equine Veterinary Science*, *57*, 29–34. https://doi.org/10.1016/j.jevs.2017.06.004

Singer, J. W., Bobsin, N., Kluchinski, D., & Bamka, W. J. (2001). Equine stocking density effect on soil chemical properties, botanical composition, and species density. *Communications in Soil Science and Plant Analysis*, 32(15–16), 2549–2559. https://doi.org/10.1081/CSS-120000390

Smith, D. G., Mayes, R. W., Hollands, T., Cuddeford, D., Yule, H. H., Malo ladrero, C. M., & Gillen, E. (2007). Validating the alkane pair technique to estimate dry matter intake in equids. *The Journal of Agricultural Science*, *145*(3), 273–281. https://doi.org/10.1017/S0021859607006788

Stewart, A. S., Pratt-Phillips, S., & Gonzalez, L. M. (2017). Alterations in intestinal permeability: The role of the "Leaky Gut" in health and disease. *Journal of Equine Veterinary Science*, *52*, 10–22. https://doi.org/10.1016/j.jevs.2017.02.009

Suagee-Bedore, J. K., Hebrock, S., Sundin, O., Lengi, A. J., Corl, B. A., & Worth, M. (2022). Thirty-two weeks of oral supplementation with LinPro™ increases hoof growth in healthy mares. *Journal of Equine Veterinary Science*, *117*, 104086. https://doi.org/10.1016/j.jevs.2022.104086

Tomlinson, D. J., Mülling, C. H., & Fakler, T. M. (2004). Invited review: Formation of keratins in the bovine claw: Roles of hormones, minerals, and vitamins in functional claw integrity. *Journal of Dairy Science*, *87*(4), 797–809. https://doi.org/10.3168/jds.S0022-0302(04)73223-3

Torfs, S., Delesalle, C., Vanschandevijl, K., De Clercq, D., Van Loon, G., Nollet, H., & Deprez, P. (2008). Anti-inflammatory phytotherapeutics: A valuable alternative to NSAID treatment in horses? *Vlaams Diergeneeskundig Tijdschrift*, *77*(3). https://doi.org/10.21825/vdt.87206

Undersander, D., Albert, B., Cosgrove, D., Johnson, D., & Peterson, P. (2002). *Pastures for profit: A guide to rotational grazing.* Cooperative Extension Publishing, University of Wisonsin-Extension.

Van der Kolk, J. H., Wijnberg, I. D., Westermann, C. M., Dorland, L., de Sain-van der Velden, M. G. M., Kranenburg, L. C., Duran, M., Dijkstra, J. A., van der Lugt, J. J., Wanders, R. J. A., & Gruys, E. (2010). Equine acquired multiple acyl-CoA dehydrogenase deficiency (MADD) in 14 horses associated with ingestion of Maple leaves (Acer pseudoplatanus) covered with European tar spot (Rhytisma acerinum). *Molecular Genetics and Metabolism*, *101*, (2–3), 289–291. doi: 10.1016/j.ymgme.2010.06.019. Epub 2010 Jul 23.

Van Soest, P. J., Robertson, J. B., & Lewis, B. A. (1991). Methods for dietary fiber, neutral detergent fiber, and nonstarch polysaccharides in relation to animal nutrition. *Journal of Dairy Science*, *74*(10), 3583–3597. https://doi.org/10.3168/jds.S0022-0302(91)78551-2

Varloud, M., Fombelle, A. de, Goachet, A. G., Drogoul, C., & Julliand, V. (2004). Partial and total apparent digestibility of dietary carbohydrates in horses as affected by the diet. *Animal Science*, *79*(1), 61–72. https://doi.org/10.1017/S1357729800054539

Vatistas, N. J., Snyder, J. R., Carlson, G., Johnson, B., Arthu, R. M., Thurmond, M., Zhou, H., & Lloyd, K. L. K. (1999). Cross-sectional study of gastric ulcers of the squamous mucosa in Thoroughbred racehorses. *Equine Veterinary Journal*, *31*(S29), 34–39. https://doi.org/10.1111/j.2042-3306.1999.tb05166.x

Verhaar, N. M. S. (2010). *Feeding practices in the sport horse industry on the North Island of New Zealand.* Massey University.

Vervuert, I., Voigt, K., Hollands, T., Cuddeford, D., & Coenen, M. (2009). Effect of feeding increasing quantities of starch on glycaemic and insulinaemic responses in healthy horses. *The Veterinary Journal*, *182*(1), 67–72. https://doi.org/10.1016/j.tvjl.2008.04.011

Vineyard, K. R., Warren, L. K., & Kivipelto, J. (2010). Effect of dietary omega-3 fatty acid source on plasma and red blood cell membrane composition and immune function in yearling horses. *Journal of Animal Science*, *88*(1), 248–257. https://doi.org/10.2527/jas.2009-2253

Volaire, F., & Lelièvre, F. (1997). Production, persistence, and water-soluble carbohydrate accumulation in 21 contrasting populations of Dactylis glomerata L. subjected to severe drought in the south of France. *Australian Journal of Agricultural Research*, *48*(7), 933. https://doi.org/10.1071/A97004

Weese, J. S., & Martin, H. (2011). Assessment of commercial probiotic bacterial contents and label accuracy. *The Canadian Veterinary Journal = La Revue Veterinaire Canadienne*, *52*(1), 43–46.

White, L. M. (1973). Carbohydrate reserves of grasses: A review. *Journal of Range Management*, *26*(1), 13. https://doi.org/10.2307/3896873

WHO International Agency for Research on Cancer. (1993). *IARC monographs on the evaluation of carcinogenic risks to humans. Some naturally occurring substances: Food items and constituents, heterocyclic aromatic amines and mycotoxins* (Vol. 56).

Wichtel, J. J., & Whitlock, R. H. (1991). Botulism associated with feeding alfalfa hay to horses. *Journal of the American Veterinary Medical Association*, *199*(4), 471–472. https://doi.org/10.2460/javma.1991.199.04.471

Williams, C. A., Kenny, L. B., & Burk, A. O. (2019). Effects of grazing system, season, and forage carbohydrates on glucose and insulin dynamics of the grazing horse. *Journal of Animal Science*, *97*(6), 2541–2554. https://doi.org/10.1093/jas/skz103

Winther, K., Kharazmi, A., Hansen, A. S. V., & Falk-Rønne, J. (2012). The absorption of natural vitamin C in horses and anti-oxidative capacity: A randomised, controlled study on trotters during a three-month intervention period. *Comparative Exercise Physiology*, *8*(3–4), 195–201. https://doi.org/10.3920/CEP12006

Wolf, P., Siesenop, U., Verspohl, J., & Kamphues, J. (2014). Hygienic quality of feedstuffs for small mammals sent to the consultation service. *Tierarztliche Praxis. Ausgabe K, Kleintiere/Heimtiere*, *42*(2), 101–106.

Woodward, M. C., Huff, N. K., Garza, F., Keowen, M. L., Kearney, M. T., & Andrews, F. M. (2014). Effect of pectin, lecithin, and antacid feed supplements (Egusin®) on gastric ulcer scores, gastric fluid pH and blood gas values in horses. *BMC Veterinary Research*, *10*(S1), S4. https://doi.org/10.1186/1746-6148-10-S1-S4

CHAPTER 3

Formulating rations for horses

Understanding and reading the feed tag or brochure is an important part of diet evaluation and formulation. Horses' dietary requirements vary depending on several factors (age, breed, metabolism, climate, activity level), and the diet is chosen to meet these requirements (Figure 3.1). Common feeding practices range from feeding traditional home cereal-based mixes to various forms of manufactured feeds. Common additions include various types of vegetable oil, succulents, one or more vitamin and mineral mixes, herbal mixes, supplements for joint health, and certain ergogenic agents with performance-enhancing claims. Dietary supplementation information is also available from several studies (Kaya-Karasu et al., 2018; Cooper & Mason, 1998; Honoré & Uhlinger, 1994), and overall, it would appear that more than 60% of horses receive a dietary supplement in the form of commercial vitamins or mineral mixtures (Figure 3.1).

There has been an assessment of supplement usage in both the US and the UK, revealing a prevalent trend in their consumption by horses (Burk & Williams, 2008; Ireland et al., 2011). Studies have reported joint supplements and electrolytes as being most widely used in the UK and US (Burk & Williams, 2008; Agar et al., 2016), but there is growth in the use of digestive aid supplements. A recent report showed that horses receiving some nutritional supplements were twice as likely to have excessive dietary levels in at least one nutritional category compared with non-supplemented horses, increasing the likelihood of an improperly balanced ration (Honoré & Uhlinger, 1994). A study that investigated the use of supplements in performance horses reported that 95% of respondents reported feeding at least one supplement. While most respondents reported adhering to manufacturers' recommended levels of feeding, over 10% reported exceeding

DOI: 10.1201/9781003379355-3

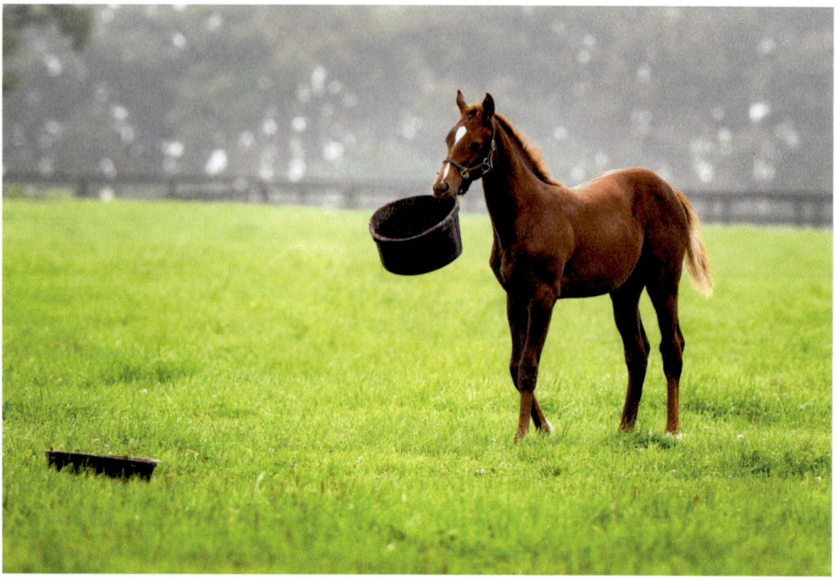

Figure 3.1 The horse's diet.

this, with most of these being in the professional sector (Agar et al., 2016). Grimwood (2016) reported that phosphorus, calcium, sodium, and potassium intakes were higher than NRC recommendations, with most estimated mineral intakes originating from the forage component of the diet. Most trainers and owners have little concept of their horses' mineral and vitamin needs and what is supplied by commercial feeds and supplements; hence, choosing supplements becomes difficult. Causes of deficiencies can include low specifications of certain nutrients in feeds and supplements and a lower intake of commercial feeds and supplements than recommended. In particular, diluting commercial feeds with straight grains or feeding lower amounts than recommended leads to lower nutrient intakes than the nutritionist intended when the feed was designed. Trainers and owners need to use commercial feed at recommended amounts; if they feed lower amounts to reduce the energy intake from the feed, they should use a more concentrated commercial feed such as a semi-concentrate or a ration balancer, or top up with a ration balancer. Using a good brand of commercial feed and supplement does not guarantee that the horses' needs are adequately met. Therefore, using feed supplements without proper guidance and education could prove detrimental to the horse (Geor et al., 2013). As a result, we will begin this section by reading the feed tag and continue with diet evaluation and formulations.

3.1 Reading the feed tag

Feed tags are attached to every bag of feed and supplements, and they contain a variety of information based on legislation. Feed tag details are additionally posted on the product website, ensuring clarity and transparency when comparing products within the equine industry. The main advantages of using feed labels include being able to compare and choose products more easily, knowing what ingredients a feed or supplement product contains, and selecting products that interest you or meet your horses' nutritional needs.

Regulation (EC) No 767/2009 of the European Parliament and of the Council of 13 July 2009 on the placing on the market and use of feed sets out general and specific labeling requirements for feed materials, compound feed, and medicated or dietetic feed for both food-producing and non-food-producing animals in Europe. The Association of American Feed Control Officials (AAFCO) is a voluntary membership organization that is comprised of personnel representing state and federal feed regulatory agencies in the US. The association is advised by industry and consumer representatives with the intent of designing feed regulations that provide fair and equitable commerce for all stakeholders. The regulations and feed laws developed by the AAFCO or European Parliament and of the Council guarantee the product you buy is safe, consistent, and meets the nutritional statements on the tag. A major function of feed regulation is to safeguard the health of humans and animals, and a critical component of that function is to ensure that animal feed and feed ingredients are appropriately and safely used as provided by the product label. Scope Regulation 767/2009, applicable as of 1 September 2010, sets out new rules for the labeling and marketing of feed and pet food. The main objective of this regulation is the harmonization and simplification of feed legislation that was previously scattered over seven directives and one decision. According to safety and marketing requirements, a feed may only be placed on the market and used if:

(a) It is safe.
(b) It does not have a direct adverse effect on the environment or animal welfare.

The information presented on an animal feed label is based on many factors, such as the intent of the product (single ingredient versus complete ration) or the species to which the product is intended to be fed. The front, back, and sides of a package are filled with information to inform us what the feed contains and provide guidance in understanding feed and making better selections for horses. "Label" means any tag, brand, mark, pictorial, or other descriptive matter written, printed, stenciled, marked, embossed, impressed on, or attached to the packaging or the container of feed (Regulation (EC), 767/2009). "Labeling" means the attribution of any words, particulars, trademarks, brand name, pictorial matter, or symbol to a feed by placing this information on any medium referring to or accompanying such feed, such as packaging, container, notice, label, document, ring, collar, or the Internet, including for advertising purposes (Regulation (EC), 767/2009).

Understanding horse feed labels is crucial for horse owners for several reasons:

1. **Proper nutrition:** Horse feed labels provide information about the composition and nutritional content of the feed. By understanding these labels, horse owners can ensure they provide their horses with a balanced and appropriate diet that meets their specific nutritional needs. This is essential for maintaining good health, supporting growth and development, and optimizing performance.
2. **Health and well-being:** Different horses have different dietary requirements based on factors such as age, breed, activity level, and health status. By reading and understanding feed labels, horse owners can select feeds that are suitable for their horse's specific needs. This helps prevent nutrient deficiencies or excesses that could lead to health issues such as weight gain/loss, metabolic disorders, or deficiencies in essential nutrients like vitamins and minerals.
3. **Ingredient identification:** Some horses find certain ingredients unpalatable and may display sensitivities to other ingredients (e.g., oats). In addition, owners may prefer to avoid certain ingredients because of poor-quality protein, risks of mycotoxin contamination (e.g., copra meal), digestibility issues, or environmental considerations (e.g., palm kernel meal). By studying the composition, you can make sure your feed doesn't contain anything you would like to avoid in a feed.
4. **Performance and training:** For performance horses, good nutrition plays a vital role in their performance. By carefully examining feed labels, horse owners can select feeds that provide the necessary protein, minerals, vitamins, and, most importantly, energy. Energy can be obtained from carbohydrates, fats, and proteins. Protein is not very efficiently utilized for energy. Carbohydrates can be classified based on their digestion process; for instance, grains, which are rich in starch, are digested by enzymes in the small intestine. On the other hand, forages and high-fiber by-products undergo fermentation in the large intestine, providing less digestible energy. Fat, with 2.25–3 times more energy than grains, is also included in feeds due to its designation as a concentrated "cool energy" source.
5. **Cost-effectiveness:** Understanding feed labels helps horse owners compare different feed options and make informed decisions based on their

budget. By knowing the nutritional content, ingredient quality, and recommended feeding amounts, horse owners can evaluate the cost-effectiveness of various feeds and select those that provide the best value for their horses' nutritional needs.

6. **Compliance with regulations:** Feed labels often include important information regarding regulatory compliance, such as batch numbers, manufacturing information, and labeling requirements. By understanding these labels, horse owners can ensure that their feed meets the necessary quality and safety standards.

In summary, understanding horse feed labels empowers horse owners to make informed decisions about their horses' nutrition, health, and overall well-being. It enables them to provide the appropriate feed that meets their horses' specific requirements, promotes optimal performance, and ensures long-term health and vitality.

The feed label

Regulation (EC), 767/2009 of the European Union establishes requirements for the labeling and composition of animal feed. According to this regulation, feed labels must include the following information:

1. **Product name:** The label should clearly indicate the name of the feed product.
2. **Ingredients:** The label should list all the ingredients used in the feed product. This includes both main ingredients and additives.
3. **Analytical constituents:** The feed label must provide information on the levels or concentrations of certain nutrients or components. These include crude protein, crude fat, crude fiber, moisture, and ash content.
4. **Additives:** If any additives are used in the feed product, the label must list them and specify their purpose or function.
5. **Instructions for use:** The label should provide guidance on the recommended usage and feeding instructions for the feed product. This may include dosage, frequency, and any specific instructions.
6. **Net weight:** The weight or quantity of the feed product should be clearly indicated on the label.
7. **Batch number/identification:** A unique batch number or identification code should be included on the label to facilitate traceability and product recall, if necessary.
8. **Manufacturer/supplier information:** The label should include the name and address of the manufacturer or supplier responsible for the feed product.
9. **Country of origin:** The label must indicate the country where the feed product was manufactured or produced.

10. **Storage conditions:** If specific storage conditions are necessary to maintain the quality and integrity of the feed product, the label should provide instructions regarding temperature, humidity, or other relevant conditions.
11. **Date of manufacture and best-before date:** This is a guide to the feed's use-by date and age.

Different regions and countries may have their own specific regulations and requirements for animal feed labeling.

According to Regulation (EC), 767/2009, the product name and purpose statement of horse feed should reflect the intended use of the feed and provide information about the type of horse being fed. The following descriptions are commonly used for horse feed products:

- **Compound feed:** A mixture of at least two feed materials, with or without feed additives, formulated for oral animal feeding. Compound feed can be in the form of complete feed or complementary feed.
- **Complete feed:** Compound feed that, due to its composition, provides all the necessary nutrients for a horse's daily ration. It is designed to be fed as the sole source of nutrition without additional forage.
- **Complementary feed:** Compound feed that has a high content of certain substances but is not sufficient to meet a horse's daily nutritional requirements on its own. Complementary feed should be combined with other feed to provide a complete diet.
- **Mineral feed:** Complementary feed that contains a minimum of 40% crude ash. Mineral feed is formulated to provide specific minerals and trace elements to supplement a horse's diet.
- **Milk replacer:** Compound feed in dry form or after dilution in liquid, used to feed foals as a complement or substitute for post-colostral milk.
- **Feed intended for particular nutritional purposes:** Feed that has a specific composition or manufacturing method, which distinguishes it from ordinary feed. This type of feed is formulated to satisfy a particular nutritional purpose, such as addressing specific health conditions or dietary needs.

These descriptions help horse owners understand the nature and purpose of the feed product, such as whether it is suitable for young horses, breeding mares, or performance horses or serves a specific nutritional purpose. These terms on the product labels provide clarity and guidance to horse owners when selecting appropriate feed for their horses.

Guaranteed analysis or nutritional analysis

The guaranteed analysis section of a horse feed label provides important information about the nutrient content and composition of the feed. It typically includes the minimum or maximum levels of various nutrients or components present in the feed. All nutrients guaranteed on the tag may be subject to testing by regulatory agencies to determine whether the tag guarantees are accurate by the AAFCO and EC (European Commission). The numbers listed in the guaranteed analysis do not provide information about the quality of the feed unless they are evaluated together with the ingredients used in the feed and the feed processing methods applied. The guaranteed analysis is a set of minimum or maximum values that will be present in the horse feed. These values are often presented as percentages. However, nutritional analysis provides a more comprehensive breakdown of the actual nutrient content of the product. It includes specific amounts of the following nutrients. Another key consideration in the analysis involves distinguishing between the dry matter (DM) and as-fed basis. The analysis may be expressed on an as-fed basis, representing the quantity present in the actual feed. On the other hand, some analyses are conducted on a DM basis, where the calculations are based on the DM content of the feed rather than its overall composition.

Below is an explanation of the key elements found in the guaranteed analysis section of horse feed labels.

Energy

In horse nutrition, different energy values are used to evaluate the energy content and utilization of feed. These energy systems include gross energy (GE), net energy (NE), digestible energy (DE), and metabolizable energy (ME) (Figure 3.2) (NRC, 2007; Geor, 2013). Each energy system is explained below (Figure 3.2).

Gross energy (GE): Gross energy represents the total energy content of a feed, including all potential energy sources. It is measured by the heat produced when the feed is burned completely. GE does not account for the energy lost during digestion and metabolism.

Digestible energy: Digestible energy refers to the portion of the GE that the horse actually digests and absorbs. It represents the energy available for the horse's use after accounting for energy losses in feces.

Metabolizable energy: Metabolizable energy represents the energy available to the horse for maintenance, growth, and activity after accounting for energy losses not only through feces but also through urine and gases produced during digestion. ME considers the energy lost in the urine and gases (methane and carbon dioxide) produced in the gastrointestinal tract. This figure is used with ruminants rather than horses in most countries.

Net energy: Net energy represents the energy available to the horse for maintenance, growth, and activity after accounting for all energy losses, including those related to digestion, metabolism, and heat increment. In the Netherlands, the energy evaluation system for horse feed diets is commonly based on the CVB (Centraal Veevoeder Bureau) system (CVB, 2005). The CVB system utilizes the concept of NE rather than DE to evaluate the

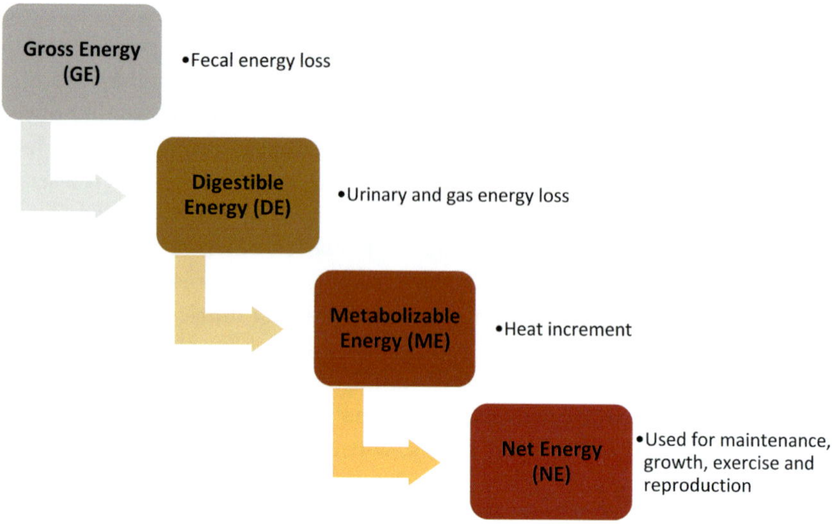

Figure 3.2 The basic partitioning of energy (adapted from NRC, 2007).

energy content of feed ingredients and formulate horse diets. The CVB system provides tables and guidelines that specify the NE values for various feed ingredients commonly used in horse diets. These NE values consider the digestibility of different nutrients and provide an estimate of the energy that can be absorbed and utilized by the horse. By using the NE values provided by the CVB system, nutritionists and horse owners in the Netherlands can calculate and formulate horse feed diets to meet the specific energy requirements of individual horses based on factors such as age, body weight, activity level, and health status.

It's important to note that the specific energy values for different feeds can vary and are typically determined through laboratory analyses and calculations based on their composition.

Current energy systems attempt to predict an individual animal's requirements (in terms of GE, DE, ME, NE, or any other unit), i.e., match supply with demand and maintain the balance shown in Table 3.1. Each system has its strengths and weaknesses, which has led to intensive and passionate discussions among scientists.

- **Crude protein (minimum):** This represents the total amount of protein in the feed and is expressed as a percentage. Protein is essential for muscle development, tissue repair, and overall growth in horses. The crude protein percentage measures the minimum total amount of protein in the feed that does not consider quality or digestibility. Protein is made up of a variety of amino acids, with certain amino acids (such as lysine, methionine,

Table 3.1 Energy systems for horses currently in use, their basis, and energy units used

Basis	*Energy unit*	*Country of use*
Digestible energy (DE)	Mcal or MJ	US, UK, Australia, Canada, Germany, Austria
Metabolizable energy (ME)	MJ	Germany
Net energy (NE)	UFC, EWpa	Netherlands, Belgium, France, Spain, Italy, Portugal

Source: adapted from Geor et al., 2013)

Mcal = megacalorie; MJ = megajoule; 1 Mcal ≈ 4.183 MJ.

UFC = French horse feed unit (NE of 1 kg DM barley; 1 UFC = 9.42 MJ NE); EWpa = Dutch equine feed unit (NE of 1 kg DM oats; 1 EWpa = 8.93 MJ NE).

DE is based on NRC 2007; ME is based on DLG 2011. In preparation, NE is based on CVB.

and threonine) required to meet your horse's nutritional needs, as well as nitrogen-containing compounds that serve as protein building blocks. The horse's total ration, including forage, should contain 10% to 14% protein, depending on their age, work discipline, and workload. Crude protein levels in horse feeds typically range from 8% to 20%, but in low-intake balancer feeds, levels can reach 30%–32%. Protein quality is more important than protein percentage, and lysine is accepted as the first-limiting amino acid for horses; requirement figures are published so that lysine level can be used in this assessment. A limiting essential amino acid means that it must come from the diet. Because of their high lysine content, soybean meal, canola/rapeseed meal, alfalfa, and green pasture are the best sources of high-quality protein, whereas most grains and hay are low in lysine (See Chapter 2, Table 2.3) (NRC, 2007).

- **Crude fat (minimum):** This indicates the total fat content in the feed and is expressed as a percentage. Fats are a concentrated energy source for horses and play a role in providing essential fatty acids and fat-soluble vitamins. Because fat contains a lot of energy, high-fat feeds are typically higher in calories. Fat is 2.25–3 times more energy-dense than carbohydrates or proteins, making it an excellent and easily digestible source of energy. High-fat feeds are popular and can benefit athletic horses, particularly racehorses, hard keepers, endurance horses, or those with certain issues such as behavior problems, myopathy, or equine gastric ulcer syndrome (EGUS). Typical horse feeds contain between 3% and 12% fat, though some specifically designed to be high-fat supplements may contain even more.
- **Crude fiber (maximum):** This represents the indigestible fiber content of the feed and is expressed as a percentage. The crude fiber percentage is a measure of the maximum percentage of fiber in the feed. Forages

are high-fiber (structural carbohydrate) feedstuffs that should be the foundation of all horse diets because horses are herbivorous and their digestive system is designed to suit a grazing lifestyle. As a result, horses should be getting enough fiber from their forage consumption. Fiber content in feed varies greatly, ranging from 6% to 30%. However, because fiber and energy are inversely related, crude fiber percentages greater than 15%–20% are relatively low in energy. In general, as the percentage of fiber decreases, the percentage of soluble carbohydrates increases. Crude fiber is a very crude estimate of the fiber content, and figures determined by analysis, such as neutral detergent fiber, give a better understanding of fiber quantity and quality in a feed.

- **Starch and non-structural carbohydrates (NSCs):** This value is particularly relevant to many athletic horses, which require starch to replenish glycogen stores or horses requiring low-NSC diets, e.g., equine metabolic syndrome (EMS). For healthy performance horses, it is often recommended not to provide more than 2 g starch/kg BW per meal (Julliand et al., 2006), although other authors have advocated 1 g starch/kg BW per meal (Geor & Harris, 2007; Julliand et al., 2006 ; Vervuert et al., 2009), as higher NSC amounts can reduce large-intestinal pH and fiber fermentation in the hindgut (Richards et al., 2006; Medina et al., 2002; Drogoul et al., 2001).
- **Ash:** Ash content refers to the mineral content of the feed and is expressed as a percentage. It includes minerals such as calcium, phosphorus, magnesium, and trace elements. Ash content helps assess the total mineral composition of the feed.
- **Moisture:** This indicates the amount of water present in the feed and is expressed as a percentage. Moisture content affects the weight and consistency of the feed, and a higher moisture content may indicate a more perishable product. The calculation of dry matter involves subtracting the moisture percentage from 100. The moisture content indicates the amount of water present in horse feed, and this factor becomes particularly notable, for example, in haylages, where moisture levels can be notably elevated. Consequently, a high moisture percentage in haylages implies that a significant proportion of the feed consists of water, emphasizing the importance of considering the actual DM nutrient concentration when assessing and purchasing horse feed.
- **Vitamins and minerals:** The vitamins and minerals section on a horse feed tag provides information about the specific vitamins and minerals present in the feed. This section is important because vitamins and minerals are essential for maintaining overall health, supporting metabolic functions, and promoting proper growth and development in horses. Some labels report added vitamins and minerals, while others report the total vitamin and mineral content. Vitamin and mineral deficiencies and excesses may cause health problems in horses (Tables 3.2 and 3.3).

Table 3.2 Minerals in Horses' Diet - Roles, Deficiency Symptoms, and Excess Symptoms

Minerals	*Role in horse's physiology*	*Deficiency symptoms*	*Excess symptoms*
Macro minerals			
Calcium (Ca)	Supports bone and tooth health, muscle contraction, blood coagulation, and the regulation of many enzymes.	Weakened skeleton and bones, dental problems, muscle spasms.	Developmental bone disorders through impact on other minerals, and maybe uroliths in some horses.
Phosphorus (P)	Works with calcium for bone and tooth health and energy production associated with ADP and ATP.	Weak bones, rachitic-like changes in growing horses, and osteomalacic changes in mature horses. Poor growth, reduced appetite.	Reduces calcium absorption rate and leads to chronic calcium deficiency and nutritional secondary hyperparathyroidism (NSH).
Magnesium (Mg)	An important ion in the blood, it activates many enzymes and participates in muscle contractions.	Nervousness, muscle tremors, and ataxia, with the potential for collapse and hyperpnea.	No controlled studies evaluating the toxicity of magnesium in horses have been done.
Potassium (K)	A major intracellular cation involved in maintenance of acid-base balance, osmotic pressure, and neuromuscular excitability.	Anorexia and, therefore, loses weight and becomes unthrifty in appearance.	The effect of excess intake has not been studied. Forages have very high levels and horses excrete K readily in the kidneys.
Sodium (Na)	A major extracellular cation and the major electrolyte involved in the maintenance of acid-base balance and osmotic regulation of body fluids.	Lack of thirst, muscle dysfunction, and unsteady gait.	Excessive thirst; will typically be excreted in the urine.

(*Continued*)

Table 3.2 (Continued) Minerals in Horses' Diet - Roles, Deficiency Symptoms, and Excess Symptoms

Minerals	*Role in horse's physiology*	*Deficiency symptoms*	*Excess symptoms*
Chlorie (Cl)	An important extracellular anion involved in acid-base balance and osmotic regulation, an essential component of bile, important in the formation of hydrochloric acid, a component of gastric secretions.	Metabolic alkalosis, decreased food intake, weight loss, muscle weakness, decreased milk production, dehydration, and constipation.	Tolerant of high concentrations.
Microminerals (trace minerals)			
Cobalt (Co)	A component of vitamin B12 involved in several important functions, e.g., red blood cell production, nervous system function, and energy metabolism.	Results in a vitamin B12 deficiency – no known cases.	Excess or toxicity in horses is rare and unlikely to occur through a natural diet.
Copper (Cu)	Essential for enzymes involved in the synthesis and maintenance of elastic connective tissue, the mobilization of iron stores, and melanin synthesis.	Coat discoloration and skeletal abnormalities, e.g., osteochondrosis, epiphysitis.	Toxicosis is rare, but features liver disease, hemolytic anemia and hemoglobinuria.
Iron (Fe)	Contained in hemoglobin, myoglobin, and many enzyme systems, and plays a critical role in oxygen transport and cellular respiration.	Microcytic, hypochromic anemia.	Especially toxic to young animals and has led to deaths among foals.

Manganese (Mn)	Essential for carbohydrate and lipid metabolism and for the synthesis of the chondroitin sulfate, which is necessary in cartilage formation.	Abnormal cartilage development; however, no direct evidence exists.	Large amounts can interfere with phosphorus absorption.
Selenium (Se)	Plays a role in immune function, in the control of thyroid hormone metabolism, and in muscle function.	Nutritional myopathy (white muscle disease), muscle weakness, impaired locomotion, and impaired immune function.	Susceptible to selenium toxicity. Acute toxicity (blind staggers) is characterized by apparent blindness. Chronic toxicity (alkali disease) is characterized by alopecia, especially about the mane and tail, and hoof defects.
Zinc (Zn)	A component of more than 100 enzymes. Plays a role in wound healing and hoof health.	Inappetence, reduced growth, alopecia, and poor wound healing and hoof quality.	Quite tolerant of excess dietary zinc; however, at very high levels, zinc reduces copper absorption.
Iodine (I)	Necessary for the synthesis of thyroid hormones, including thyroxine (T4) and triiodothyronine (T3).	Hypothyroidism resulting in thyroid gland hypertrophy or goiter.	Toxicity occurs only when iodine is oversupplemented or when animals are receiving feeds containing unusually high amounts of iodine, such as some types of seaweed.

Source: Adapted from NRC, 2007

Table 3.3 Vitamins in horses' diet – roles, deficiency symptoms, and excess symptoms

Vitamins	*Role in horse's physiology*	*Deficiency symptoms*	*Excess symptoms*
Fat-soluble vitamins			
Vitamin A	Plays a role in night vision, crucial roles in reproduction and embryogenesis, and is important for maintaining the immune response.	Night blindness, poor reproduction, weakened immune system, and reduced growth.	Bone fragility, implicated in DOD.
Vitamin D	Important role in calcium homeostasis, bone health.	Rickets, a disease characterized by bone deformities.	Toxicity is associated with calcification of soft tissue and death.
Vitamin E	Biological, antioxidant, muscle function, and immune support.	White muscle disease in foals, equine degenerative myeloencephalopathy (EDM) in young horses, equine motor neuron disease (EMND), muscle weakness, poor immune function, and nerve damage.	Does not appear to be toxic to horses.
Vitamin K	Blood clotting and bone metabolism.	Impaired blood clotting, increased bleeding tendencies, and problems with bone health and integrity.	Interference with blood-thinning medications.
Water-soluble vitamins			
Vitamin B1 (thiamine)	Involved in carbohydrate and energy metabolism	Anorexia, bradycardia, muscle fasciculations, and ataxia.	Has not been reported in horses

Vitamin B2 (riboflavin)	Involved in lipid metabolism and antioxidant defense mechanisms.	Has not been described in horses; signs in other species include rough hair coat and dermatitis.	Little evidence exists of oral toxicity.
Vitamin B3 (niacin)	Involved in many important biological oxidation-reduction reactions.	Has not been described in the horses.	Has not been described in horses.
Vitamin B7 (biotin)	Important role in intermediary metabolism and essential for cell proliferation.	Poor hoof quality, such as soft white line and crumbling and fissured horn at the bearing border of the hoof wall.	Has not been described in horses.
Vitamin B12 (cobalamin)	A component of several enzyme systems involved in protein synthesis, and carbohydrate and fat metabolism.	No evidence of vitamin B12 deficiency has been seen.	Has not been described in horses.
Vitamin C (ascorbic acid)	A biological antioxidant involved in the synthesis of collagen and carnitine.	No evidence of vitamin C deficiency has been seen.	Has not been described in horses.

Source: adapted from NRC, 2007

Minerals: The guaranteed or nutritional analysis includes information about the levels of macro- and microminerals.

Macrominerals: Macrominerals are indispensable components that play diverse and vital roles in maintaining the overall health and functionality of the horse body. The main roles are:

- Essential for the structural integrity of bones and teeth, macrominerals play a crucial role in supporting the framework of the body.
- Macrominerals are necessary to maintain the body's acid-base balance and fluid equilibrium, ensuring optimal physiological function.
- Macrominerals facilitate nerve conduction, contributing to the transmission of signals between nerve cells and aiding in efficient communication within the nervous system.
- Integral to muscle contraction, macrominerals are vital for the proper functioning of muscles, enabling movements and physical activities.

Calcium (Ca) and phosphorus (P) (min and max values as %): Calcium is a macromineral needed for bone metabolism, and about 99 percent of the calcium in the body is found in the bones and teeth. Ca is often expressed as a guaranteed minimum and maximum percentage of total feed. Calcium present in the bloodstream exists in three distinct forms: in a free or ionized state, in a complexed or chelated state, and bound to proteins.

- Reduced levels of ionized calcium in the blood trigger a series of responses: it stimulates the secretion of parathyroid hormone (PTH), which, in turn, prompts the synthesis of 1,25-dihydroxyvitamin D3 (1,25(OH)2D3) in the kidneys. Subsequently, 1,25(OH)2D3 facilitates the absorption of calcium in the gut and, working in conjunction with PTH, stimulates the process of bone resorption to maintain levels of calcium in the blood in a steady state. PTH also induces phosphaturia, leading to the excretion of phosphorus in the urine.

Elevated levels of ionized calcium initiate a distinct set of responses: the secretion of calcitonin is stimulated, which notably does not trigger the production of 1,25(OH)2D3. Consequently, the kidneys produce 24,25-dihydroxycholecalciferol. Subsequently, there is no stimulation of calcium absorption in the gut or bone, increased renal calcium excretion occurs, and calcitonin functions to decrease osteoclastic activity, playing a role in regulating bone density.

Calcium works in conjunction with phosphorus, so the ratio of these two minerals to one another is critical. There is no benefit to the mechanical properties of bone when the Ca supply in the diet exceeds requirements. Phosphorus is a major constituent of bone, making up 14% to 17% of the skeleton (El Shorafa et al., 1979). In addition, it is required for many energy transfer reactions associated with adenosine diphosphate (ADP) and adenosine triphosphate (ATP), and for the synthesis of phospholipids, nucleic acids, and phosphoproteins (NRC, 2007). Calcium levels should always exceed phosphorus levels in the diet, and ideally, your horse's total calcium-to-phosphorus ratio should be between 1:5 and 2:1. Calcium carbonate and dicalcium phosphate are common inorganic forms of calcium (Highfill et al., 2005) in feeds or diets for horses.

Magnesium (Mg): Magnesium plays a pivotal role primarily in bone growth and maintenance, making it the third-largest mineral constituent in bones, following calcium and phosphorus. Beyond its involvement in skeletal health, magnesium is crucial for the metabolism of carbohydrates (CHO) and lipids and for neuromuscular stability. The kidney plays a critical role in maintaining magnesium homeostasis, efficiently excreting any excess magnesium requirements through urine. The primary site for magnesium absorption is the small intestine, where it is absorbed into the bloodstream. Notably, magnesium is naturally present in most feedstuffs for horses, derived from both forages and grains, ensuring that horses receive a consistent supply of this essential mineral in their diet.

Sodium (Na), chloride (Cl), and potassium (K): These minerals play a vital role as electrolytes in maintaining fluid equilibrium within the horse's body and facilitating nerve and muscle functions.

- Sodium is essential for nerve functionality, muscle contraction, thirst, and fluid balance maintenance.
- Potassium is required for nerve and muscle function and helps to maintain sodium levels in balance.
- Chloride works with sodium and potassium to maintain proper fluid balance.

Sweating can cause electrolyte loss in horses, especially during exercise, travel, or in hot and humid climates. It is critical to replenish these electrolytes to protect the health of horses. Most of the Na and Cl appearing in sweat comes from the extracellular fluid compartment, while most of the K and some of the Cl arise from the intracellular fluid compartment (Figure 3.3). Cl is the predominant ion lost in sweat, followed by Na, and horse sweat is hypertonic. Sweat Cl losses are nearly equal to the combined losses of all cations. K is the predominant cation present in muscle and Cl is the predominant anion; both contribute to muscle osmolality and fluid volume. Thus, K lost from muscle (and nerves) needs to be replaced to restore intracellular K and muscle intracellular volume if muscle function is to be maintained at optimum levels (Lindinger & Cairns, 2021). Therefore, K ingested as part of electrolyte supplements or from forages is important to replace K within cells. In contrast, Na is primarily retained within the extracellular fluid compartment, where is it needed. Ingested electrolytes

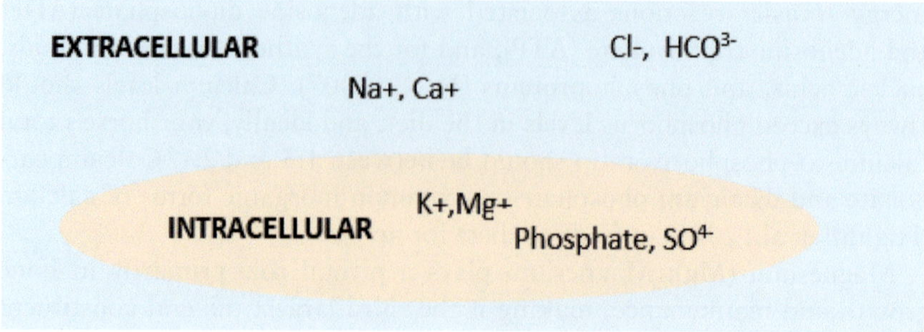

Figure 3.3 The major cations and anions found in horse body fluid.

and water are used, in part, to produce sweat and, in part, to replace water and ions that may have been lost from extra- and intracellular fluid compartments (Lindinger, 2022). Increased plasma sodium is a trigger for thirst (Figure 3.3).

In the fluids of a horse's body, electrolytes, including major cations and anions, are substances that dissolve into ions in a solution. These ions, categorized into positively charged cations (+) and negatively charged anions (–), are abundant in both intracellular fluid (ICF) and extracellular fluid (ECF). The concentration of electrolytes varies between the intracellular and extracellular environments.

Electrolyte supplementation is most beneficial for electrolyte balance, and the effectiveness of this approach varies depending on the horse's exercise. It is critical to carefully examine the label of commercial electrolyte products, as many electrolyte supplements have lower concentrations due to added sugar or vitamins (Kronfeld, 2001; Lindinger, 2022).

- **Short-duration exercise:** When the horse is dehydrated from prior transport (30 minutes or longer on warm days) or has had no access to water for more than 1 hour, then electrolyte supplementation should be administered 1 hour prior to even short-term exercise.
- **Long-duration exercise:** Long-duration exercise can be considered any form of activity where there are intentional rest periods during the activity, such as in the cross-country phase of eventing and endurance rides. Take every opportunity to provide electrolyte supplementation and ensure the horse has access to adequate amounts of cool, clean water during the ride: offer water at every rest break.

Trace minerals (minimum as parts per million or mg/kg): Copper, zinc, and selenium are among the trace minerals listed in the guaranteed analysis.

- **Copper (Cu):** Copper assumes a vital role in bone maintenance and hemoglobin function within the body. Cu is also needed for synthesizing and maintaining elastic connective tissue, mobilizing of iron stores, preserving mitochondrial integrity, synthesizing melanin, and detoxifying superoxides. While the specific copper requirements for horses have not been precisely established, it is recognized that copper is essential for sustaining healthy bones and facilitating proper hemoglobin function, which is crucial for oxygen transport in the blood. In the case of foals, their copper supply is primarily from liver stores accumulated during pregnancy, emphasizing the significance of maternal nutrition in providing essential elements for the optimal development of the offspring. The intricate interplay of copper in tendons, ligaments, bone health, and hemoglobin function underscores its importance in supporting fundamental physiological processes in horses, particularly during growth and development.
- **Zinc (Zn):** Zinc is a mineral with diverse biological roles and acts as a constituent or activator for over 100 enzymes, including many metalloenzymes such as carbonic anhydrase, alkaline phosphatase, and carboxypeptidase. Its primary functions encompass a range of critical processes, including carbohydrate metabolism, protein synthesis, hoof, skin, and wound healing, as well as playing integral roles in growth and reproduction. Zinc's influence extends to hormone production, particularly affecting testosterone, adrenal corticosteroids, and insulin. Maintaining zinc homeostasis is essential, achieved through a delicate balance of absorption, primarily occurring in the small intestine, and excretion, primarily through feces. Zinc absorption is subject to modulation by various dietary components; for instance, phytate, commonly found in certain foods, can decrease zinc absorption. Conversely, the amino acid methionine and organic acid citrate have been observed to enhance zinc absorption. This intricate interplay highlights the multifaceted role of zinc in supporting enzymatic functions and physiological processes critical for overall health and well-being.
- **Manganese (Mn):** Manganese, a trace mineral essential for equine health, is required for a variety of bodily functions. It is essential for maintaining healthy skin and coat, supporting reproductive processes, and promoting the development of fetal skeletal structures. Manganese plays an important role in the metabolism of carbohydrates and fats, as well as the synthesis of chondroitin sulfate, which is required for cartilage formation. It also serves as a component of superoxide dismutase, an antioxidant that protects against free radical damage. Manganese concentrations in forage and grains depend on soil manganese levels, which may vary.
- **Iron (Fe):** Iron is needed for hemoglobin, myoglobin, and many enzyme processes. It plays a critical role in oxygen transport and energy

production in cells. Forages, by-products like beet pulp, and soil contain high to very high levels of iron, and it is likely that most horses exceed their requirements from these sources alone. However, iron is also added to many commercial feeds and mineral supplements. Some researchers have suggested that iron may interfere with the absorption and metabolism of other minerals, such as zinc and copper. In one study, high iron intake reduced serum and liver zinc concentrations (Lawrence, 1987). However, in many studies conducted at Kentucky Equine Research, there has been no evidence that typical intakes of iron affect the digestibility of any mineral (Pagan, 2001).

- **Selenium (Se):** Selenium is needed for the selenium-dependent antioxidant glutathione peroxidase and is also involved in thyroid hormone metabolism regulation. Many areas of the world are selenium deficient, so forages and grains grown there will have low levels of selenium. Thus, horses require supplementation in feeds or supplements. However, other areas grow forages with high selenium levels, and toxicity can result. Selenium has the narrowest safety margin between requirements and toxicity.
- **Iodine (I):** Iodine is crucial for the synthesis of thyroxine (T4) and triiodothyronine (T3), both of which constitute essential thyroid hormones that regulate basal metabolism. The production of adequate thyroid hormones fails in cases of iodine deficiency. An excess of iodine, on the other hand, can directly limit thyroid hormone synthesis and release. Both cases result in increased production of thyroid-stimulating hormone (TSH), which leads to thyroid gland enlargement, a condition known as goiter.
- **Chromium (Cr) and cobalt (Co):** Chromium and cobalt are two additional trace minerals that may be listed on the feed tag. These trace minerals are frequently listed as minimum values on feed tags, with the unit "ppm" being used. An abbreviation for "parts per million," or one part for every million parts, 1 ppm is 1 mg/kg.

Vitamins

Vitamins are classified into two types: fat-soluble compounds (vitamins A, E, D, and K) and water-soluble compounds (B-complex vitamins, vitamin C). The majority of these vitamins are added to most commercial horse feeds. Fat-soluble vitamins accumulate in adipose tissue, and vitamins A and D can reach toxic levels if consumed in excess. However, deficiencies in vitamins A, E, and K have been observed. Under normal circumstances, horses can synthesize vitamins B and K within their bodies through synthesis in the gut by the microbiota, and they can produce vitamin C in the liver from glucose. Deficiencies in these vitamins are uncommon and typically occur only in specific and unusual circumstances, usually when a horse has a particular health problem. Imbalances in their levels, whether deficient or excessive, can lead to health issues, as outlined in Table 3.3.

Fat-soluble vitamins

Vitamin A is an essential nutrient with diverse functions in the body. Its primary responsibility lies in supporting vision, where it plays a key role in maintaining rhodopsin, a light-sensitive receptor in the eyes. Beyond vision, vitamin A contributes to the overall health of various body systems, influencing growth, reproduction, and immune response. In the case of horses, vitamin A is obtained in the form of pro-vitamins, particularly beta-carotene. Green-colored plants, such as fresh green forages and high-quality young hay, are rich sources of beta-carotene for horses. It is worth noting that hay storage can impact vitamin A and E levels; stored hay gradually loses these essential vitamins each month, so hay older than six months old will have low levels. This emphasizes the importance of providing horses access to fresh and high-quality forages to ensure they receive an adequate supply of vitamin A for optimal health and functioning of various physiological processes.

Vitamin D regulates calcium homeostasis within the body. It increases intestinal calcium absorption, ensuring that this essential mineral is absorbed efficiently from the digestive tract. Vitamin D also stimulates renal reabsorption, which involves both calcium and phosphorus and is regulated by parathyroid hormone. Vitamin D helps build up the bone matrix, which contributes significantly to bone health. It is essential for the calcification of osteoblasts, the cells that form bone. Vitamin D3, a basic form of vitamin D, undergoes a sequential conversion process in the body (Figure 3.4). Although vitamin D plays a role in immunity, its impact on health and disease remains unclear (Hymøller & Jensen, 2015). Horses can get vitamin D from a variety of sources, including sunlight, which is a natural source of vitamin D for animals, but is relatively ineffective in horses (Dosi et al., 2020). Horses can also get vitamin D2 from dried plant material in their diets. However, levels may vary depending on UV exposure, time since cutting, and the leaf-to-stem ratio in the plant material. In general, leafy materials contain more vitamin D. Overall, the biochemistry of vitamin D in horses is unique and poorly understood (Figure 3.4).

Vitamin E encompasses a group of compounds classified into saturated tocopherols (α, β, γ, δ) and unsaturated tocotrienols (α, β, γ, δ). In horses, vitamin E plays crucial roles, with multifaceted contributions to their well-being. It acts as an antioxidant in conjunction with selenium-containing enzymes such as glutathione peroxidase and other enzymes. Vitamin E can partially compensate for low levels of selenium. This antioxidant activity helps protect cells from oxidative damage. Beyond its role as an antioxidant, vitamin E is essential for DNA synthesis, contributing to the integrity of genetic material and cellular processes. Additionally, it serves as a cofactor for synthesizing vitamin C, further supporting the horse's overall immune function. Another notable function is its ability to enhance the absorption of vitamin A, highlighting the interconnected roles of different

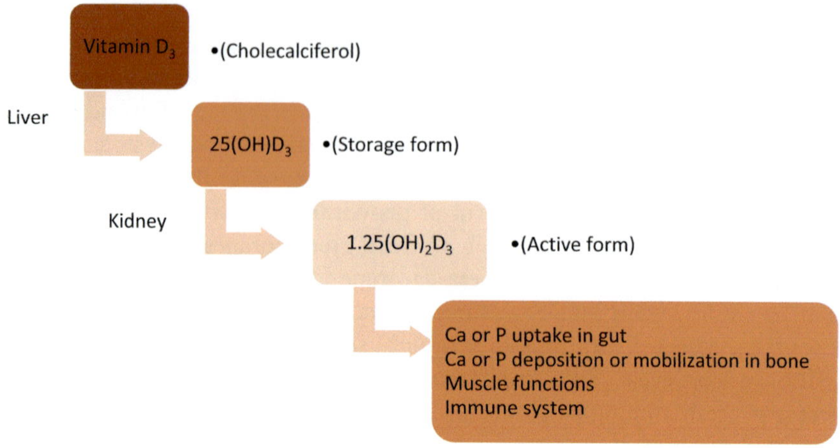

Figure 3.4 The metabolic activation of vitamin D. In the liver, it transforms into 25-hydroxyvitamin D3 (25 D3), serving as a storage form. Subsequently, in the kidney, it undergoes further conversion to its active form, 1,25-dihydroxyvitamin D3 (1.25 D3). This active form of vitamin D3 plays pivotal roles in several physiological processes, such as Ca or P deposition or mobilization in bone.

vitamins in maintaining optimal health for horses. Overall, vitamin E's diverse functions underscore its importance in supporting various physiological processes essential for the well-being of horses. Vitamin E for horses includes natural RRR-α-tocopherol acetate and synthetic dl-α-tocopherol acetate. The natural form, RRR-α-tocopherol acetate, is more biologically active. It's worth noting that the vitamin E content in forages can vary based on factors such as the maturity of the plant. Young green grass tends to have higher vitamin E levels than mature herbage. Additionally, within the plant, leaves generally contain higher levels of vitamin E than stems. Another consideration is the impact of ensilage on vitamin E levels. During the ensilage process, there may be losses in vitamin E content. Therefore, the storage and processing of forages can influence the overall vitamin E availability in a horse's diet. Like vitamin A, levels of vitamin E decline with age of the hay so more attention must be paid to supplementary vitamin E when feeding older hay. Horses that do not get regular access to green grass in their diet may require vitamin E supplementation, particularly performance horses and mares, which have higher requirements.

Vitamin K plays a crucial role in various physiological processes, particularly in the liver, where it is responsible for the carboxylation or activation of clotting factors. This function is essential for proper blood coagulation.

Additionally, vitamin K significantly impacts bone health, being vital for bone mineralization and influencing both bone formation and resorption. Numerous vitamin K-dependent proteins, such as "osteocalcin," contribute to bone health. Osteocalcin plays a key role in bone mineralization. There are three primary types of vitamin K:

- K1 (phylloquinone): Originating from plants, K1 is found in green pastures and is less abundant in dried forages. The absorption rate of K1 is relatively low, approximately 12%.
- K2 (menaquinone): Synthesized by hindgut microflora, K2 is another form of vitamin K. It plays a vital role in bone health.
- K3 (menadione): K3 is a synthetic form of vitamin K commonly supplemented in the diet. It is converted into menaquinone-4 (K2-4) in the body.

Water-soluble vitamins

Water-soluble vitamins, which include the B-complex vitamins and vitamin C, are not stored in the horse's body.

B-complex vitamins encompass thiamine (B1), riboflavin (B2), niacin (B3), pantothenic acid (B5), pyridoxine (B6), biotin (B7), folic acid (B9), and cobalamin (B12). The microbiota in the large intestine produces B vitamins; however, absorption and availability to the horse are not well studied. While supplementation of B vitamins may not be necessary for a horse with a healthy digestive tract, horses often face microbiota issues due to high-starch and low-forage diets, making B-vitamin supplementation advisable in performance horses.

Vitamin C (ascorbic acid) is synthesized in the liver from glucose within the body. Since supplemental vitamin C is not efficiently absorbed by the horse's intestine, feeding higher levels or injectable forms becomes necessary to impact blood levels. Vitamin C is an organic compound called lactone, a sugar acid derived from gluonic acid synthesized from the glucose molecule. Vitamins C and E are part of the main non-enzymatic antioxidants and are very involved in immune function (Garcia et al., 2022).

The table provides information on the various vitamins found in a horse's diet, including roles in the body, deficiency symptoms when there is an inadequate intake, and potential symptoms that may occur with excessive intake. However, it is wise to note that the specific symptoms and optimal levels of vitamins can vary based on individual horse needs, so consulting with an equine nutritionist is important for accurate assessment and guidance for a balanced diet.

Understanding the feed tag's ingredient list

Understanding the ingredient list on your horse's feed is essential for ensuring their proper nutrition. The order of ingredients is listed in descending order of inclusion, starting with the ingredient present in the highest amount. This helps you grasp the relative proportions of various components in the feed. Here is a guide to interpreting the ingredient list:

- **Specific names:** Each ingredient is listed using specific names like "oats," "corn," or "soybean meal" rather than generic terms like grains or proteins. This clarity ensures you know exactly what your horse is consuming.
- **Blended ingredients:** If the feed contains blended ingredients, each one is listed separately. For example, if it includes a mixture of grains (e.g., corn, barley, oats), each grain is specified individually.
- **Processing methods:** Specific forms or processing methods are mentioned when relevant. For instance, if the feed contains "cracked corn" or "extruded soybeans," these terms are included to provide more detailed information.
- **Generic terms:** Generic or vague descriptions like "by-products" should be avoided. Instead, specific by-products should be listed, such as "wheat bran," "wheat midds," or "rice bran."
- **Additives or supplements:** Specific additives or supplements like vitamins, minerals, probiotics, and other nutritional supplements are listed separately if present in the feed.
- **Oil:** The origin of the oil should be listed (e.g., soybean oil or linseed oil).
- **Toxic ingredients:** Some horse owners still use feeds made for other animals, and an ingredient list can help you identify toxic or undesirable components such as antibiotics or ionophores.

By paying attention to the ingredient list, the horse owner can make informed decisions about their horse's nutrition and better understand the composition of their feed.

3.2 Diet evaluation and formulation for horses

Practical diet evaluation and formulation for horses

Formulating a diet for horses requires considering several factors, including their age, weight, activity level, body condition, and specific nutritional needs. While it's always recommended to consult with an equine nutritionist for an individualized diet plan, here are some general guidelines to consider:

Evaluating and formulating a horse's diet involves several key steps to ensure their nutritional needs are met. The general steps involved in horse diet evaluation and formulation:

a. **Assess the horse's requirements:** Evaluate the specific needs of the horse based on factors such as age, breed, weight, body condition, metabolism, activity level, and overall health. Consider the horse's energy requirements, protein needs, mineral and vitamin requirements, and any special dietary considerations.
b. **Analyze current diet:** Analyze the horse's current diet, including forage (hay, pasture) and concentrates (grains, pellets, supplements). Determine the nutrient content of each component, including protein, energy, fiber, vitamins, and minerals. This can be done through laboratory analysis or using nutrient databases.
c. **Identify nutritional gaps:** Identifying nutritional gaps in a horse's diet involves comparing the nutrient requirements of the horse with the actual nutrient content of the diet. Identify any deficiencies or excesses in nutrients to ensure a balanced diet. This is easier if you use one of the commercial diet evaluation software programs, but it can be done with a spreadsheet.
d. **Select forage source:** Choose appropriate forage sources based on the horse's needs and the availability and quality of the forage. Consider factors such as nutrient content and digestibility.
e. **Select concentrate feed:** Select suitable concentrate feeds, such as grains or commercial horse feeds, to supplement the forage and meet any nutrient deficiencies. Consider the nutrient composition, palatability, and digestibility of concentrate options.
f. **Balance nutrient intake:** Calculate and adjust the amounts of forage and concentrate feeds to ensure they meet the horse's nutrient requirements. Balance the diet for energy, protein, vitamins, and minerals, avoiding both deficiencies and excesses.
g. **Monitor and adjust:** Regularly monitor the horse's weight, body condition, overall health, and performance. Make necessary adjustments to the diet based on changes in the horse's requirements, activity level, or health status.

Each horse is unique, and the diet formulation should be tailored to their individual requirements. Regular evaluation and adjustments are essential to maintain optimal health and performance. Consider any specific dietary needs the horse may have, such as allergies, metabolic conditions (e.g., insulin dysregulation), or performance requirements. Adjust the diet accordingly to accommodate these special considerations. For complex dietary needs or specific health concerns, consulting with an equine nutritionist or a veterinarian specializing in equine nutrition to ensure the diet is appropriately formulated is recommended.

Step-by-step ration calculation for horses

The step-by-step ration calculation for horses is explained below and summarized with an example in Table 3.4.

Table 3.4 Example of ration evaluation and formulation for horses

Steps	*Guideline*	*Example*
Step 1: Estimate body weight (BW)	Weight tape or digital scale.	BW = 500 kg.
Step 2: Estimate body condition score (BCS)	The BCS is commonly assessed using both the five-point system and the nine-point system for horses.	BCS 5/9.
Step 3: Predict voluntary feed intake	Typically estimated to be around 2%–3% of their body weight (as fed) per day.	If 2% feed intake = 10 kg feed per day.
Step 4: Calculate digestible energy requirement	Energy requirement for maintenance (NRC, 2007) DE (Mcal/day) = 1.4 + (0.03 x BW in kg). To convert to MJ/day, use the conversion Mcal/day × 4.183. When determining the energy requirements of exercising horses, it is important to incorporate the appropriate multiplication factor.	Maintenance energy requirement = 1.4 + (0.03 × 500) = 16.4 Mcal/day = 16.4 × 4.183 = 68.6 MJ per day. For showjumping, the multiplication factor is 1.5. DE (Mcal/d) = (0.0333 × BW) × 1.5 DE (Mcal/d) = (0.0333 × 500) × 1.5 = 24.9 Mcal/d. DE MJ per day = Mcal × 4.183 = 104 MJ.
Step 5: Calculate energy intake	Total energy intake from forage plus energy intake from concentrate feed.	Diet of horse: 9 kg of hay (forage) with an energy content of 9 MJ/kg, and 2 kg of concentrate feed with an energy content of 14 MJ/kg. Energy intake from forage = 9 kg x 9 MJ/kg = 72 MJ/day. Energy intake from concentrate feed = 2 kg x 14 MJ/kg = 28 MJ/day. Total energy intake = 81 MJ/day (forage) + 28 MJ/day (concentrate feed) = 109 MJ/day.

Table 3.4 (Continued) Example of ration evaluation and formulation for horses

Steps	*Guideline*	*Example*
Step 6: Calculate minimum forage requirement	The minimum forage intake is determined by multiplying the body weight of the horse by 1.5%, resulting in the horse's minimum DM requirement.	This translates to a minimum DM requirement of 7.5 kg of forage for a 500-kg horse.
Step 7: Calculate forage intake and choose appropriate forage	Forage intake and requirements should always be compared on a DM basis to account for lower DM/higher water content in pastures and haylages.	If the hay being fed has a DM content of 90%, then the equivalent amount would be 8.3 kg as-fed. Therefore, 9 kg of hay consumed meets the horse's minimum DM forage requirements.
Step 8: Calculate and determine the appropriate forage-to-concentrate ratio in the diet and choose concentrate sources	The ratio is calculated as the ratio of forage intake (kg/day) to concentrate intake (kg/day)	The forage-to-concentrate ratio for a diet of 9 kg hay and 2 kg concentrate is approximately 82:18. This ratio is acceptable.
Step 9: Evaluate nutrient intake and balance the ration	To ensure that the requirements are met, the diet should be evaluated for protein, starch and sugar, and vitamins and minerals.	Starch intake should be limited to no more than 2 g starch per kg BW per meal; in this case, that is 1000 g starch per meal. If the concentrate is less than 50% starch, the 2 kg of concentrate feed can be fed in one meal.

Step 1: Estimate body weight

Estimating the horses' body weight can be accomplished using different methods, depending on the conditions at the horse yard. One common method involves using weight tape specifically designed for horses, which provides a quick estimation of body weight. By placing the tape around the horse's girth, just behind the withers, the measurement on the tape can be read to estimate the weight (Figure 3.5). Additionally, several weight

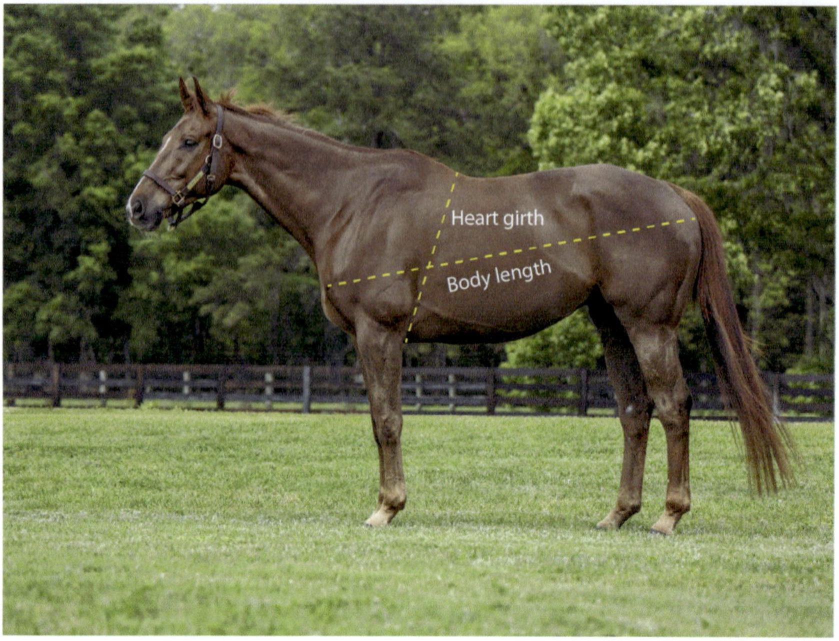

Figure 3.5 Measuring the horse's heart girth and body length to estimate body weight. Courtesy of Kentucky Equine Research.

estimation formulas have been developed based on measurements such as body length, heart girth, and cannon bone circumference. When these formulas are applied correctly, they can provide reasonably accurate estimates of body weight.

$$\text{Weight(kg) adult horses} = \frac{(\text{heart girth}^2 \times \text{body length})}{11{,}880\ \text{cm}^3}$$

This is the most accurate estimate as reported by Carroll & Huntington (1988).

Utilizing a large animal or equine-specific digital scale is the recommended approach for the most precise determination of a horse's body weight. This entails physically weighing the horse by leading it onto the scale, which offers the highest level of accuracy.

Step 2: Evaluate body condition score

Body condition scoring (BCS) is a widely used method to assess horses' body condition. It is a subjective evaluation based on a visual and tactile assessment of certain areas of the horse's body, particularly the ribs, loin,

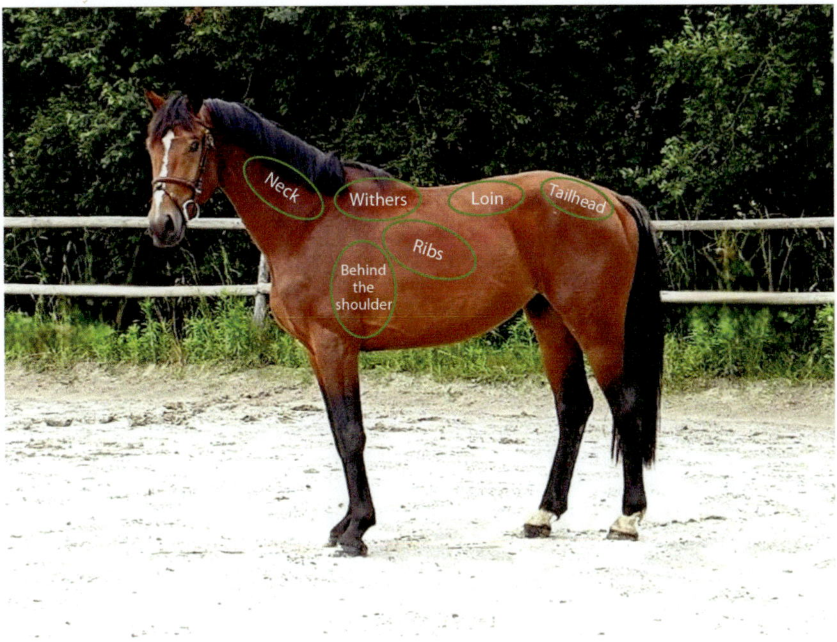

Figure 3.6 Areas to evaluate body condition score on horses.

tailhead, withers, and neck (Figure 3.6). BCS indicates the horse's overall fat cover, which is important for determining its nutritional status and health.

The five-point BCS system for horses is a simplified version of the BCS scale that assesses the fat cover of horses (Carroll & Huntington, 1988). This system categorizes body condition into five main categories, allowing for a more generalized evaluation (Table 3.5). Half scores are used.

Another study by Henneke et al. introduced the widely adopted Henneke Body Condition Scoring System for horses, which has been used extensively in the equine industry for assessing body condition. The BCS scale typically ranges from 1 to 9, with BCS 1 being extremely emaciated and BCS 9 being extremely obese (Henneke et al., 1983) (Table 3.6). The ideal body condition for most horses is generally considered to be around 5 or 6 on the scale. However, the ideal range may vary depending on the breed, age, and specific use of the horse.

It's important to regularly assess a horse's body condition to ensure proper feeding and management. The appropriate body condition will depend on the horse's individual needs, health, and intended use. Consulting with a veterinarian or equine nutritionist can provide more guidance on maintaining a healthy body condition for horses.

Table 3.5 The five-point BCS system for horses

BCS	*Explanation*
BCS 1	**Poor:** Horses with ewe neck, sunken rump, cavity under tail, ribs easily visible, pelvis and croup well defined, and deep depression under tail.
BCS 2	**Moderate:** Horses with narrow but firm neck, ribs just visible, backbone well covered, flat rump both sides of the backbone, and slight cavity under tail.
BCS 3	**Good:** Horses with a good body condition score have a firm neck and no crest, except stallions, ribs just covered but easily felt. No gutter along back, rounded rump, but pelvis easily felt. This category represents an ideal body condition for most horses.
BCS 4	**Fat:** Horses with a fat body condition score have a wide and firm neck with a crest, ribs well covered, well-rounded rump, gutter along back and rump, and pelvis hard to feel.
BCS 5	**Very fat:** Horses with an obese body condition have excessive fat deposits throughout their body. Horses with marked crest, very wide and firm neck, ribs buried and cannot be felt, deep gutter along back and rump, pelvis buried and cannot be felt.

Source: Carroll & Huntington, 1988

Step 3: Predict voluntary feed intake

The voluntary feed intake (VFI) of horses can vary depending on several factors, including the horse's size, age, breed, physiological state, diet composition, and environmental conditions. On average, horses' VFI (as fed) is typically estimated to be around 1.5%–3% of their body weight per day. However, it's important to note that individual variations and specific circumstances can cause deviations from this average range. Hard-working horses, lactating mares, and weanlings have the highest VFI.

Step 4: Calculate DE requirement

To accurately estimate the energy requirements of exercising horses, it is essential to consider the NRC multiplication factors specific to the workload intensity (Table 3.7). These factors should be included in the calculations to ensure an appropriate energy intake for the horse's exercise level.

Step 5: Calculate the energy intake

To calculate the energy intake of a horse fed a combination of forage and concentrate feed, you will need to estimate the energy content of each component and determine the appropriate proportions and intakes of each in the horse's diet. The first step is weighing the feed, as not all dippers/scoops hold 1 kg.

Calculate the energy intake from forage:

- Multiply the weight of forage consumed per day by the energy content of the forage (DE per kilogram) to obtain the daily energy intake from forage.

Calculate the energy intake from concentrate feed:

- Multiply the weight of concentrate feed consumed per day by the energy content of the concentrate feed (DE per kilogram) to obtain the daily energy intake from concentrate feed.

Sum the energy intake from forage and concentrate feed to obtain the total energy intake.

Table 3.6 The nine-point BCS system for horses

BCS	*Explanation*	
BCS 1	**Poor:** Animal extremely emaciated; spine, ribs, tailhead, points of hip, and buttock projecting prominently; bone structure of withers, shoulder, and neck easily noticeable; no fatty tissue can be felt.	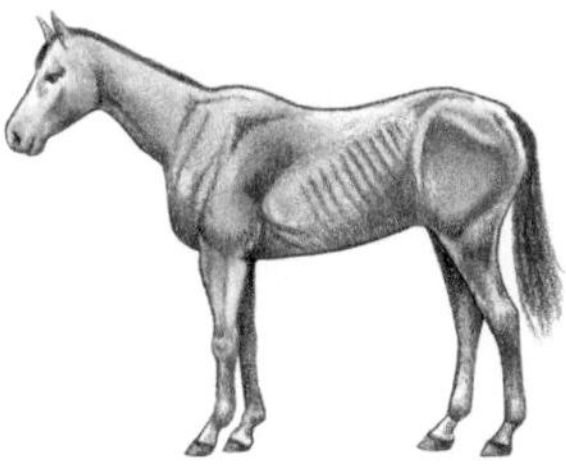
BCS 2	**Very thin:** Animal emaciated; slight fat covering over base of spine, ribs, tailhead; points of hip and buttock prominent; withers, shoulder, and neck structure faintly discernable.	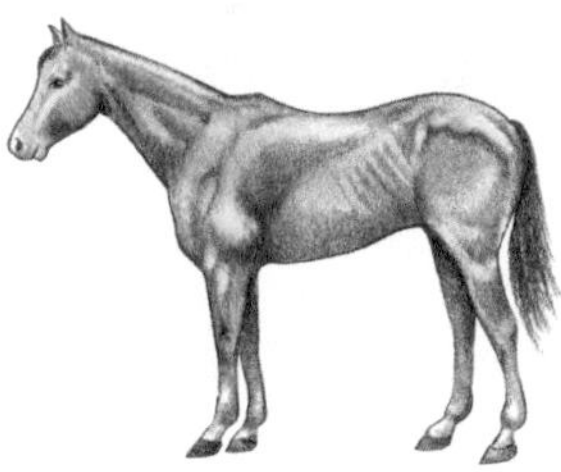
BCS 3	**Thin:** Fat buildup about halfway on spine; slight fat cover over ribs; spine and ribs easily discernable; tailhead prominent, but individual vertebrae cannot be identified visually; points of hip appear rounded but easily discernable; points of buttock not distinguishable; withers, shoulders, and neck accentuated.	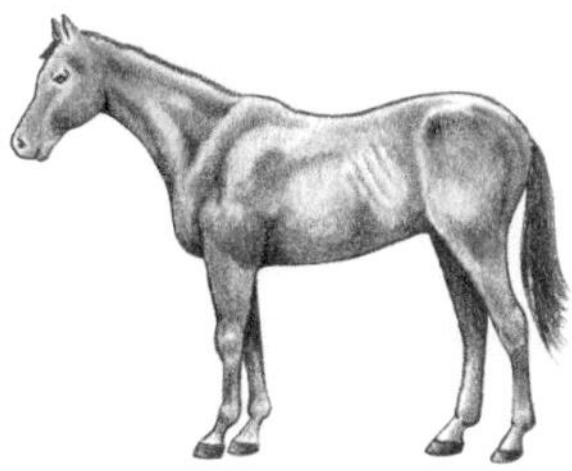

(*Continued*)

Table 3.6 (Continued) The nine-point BCS system for horses

BCS	*Explanation*	
BCS 4	**Moderately thin:** Slight ridge along back; faint outline of ribs discernable; tailhead prominence depends on conformation, fat can be felt around it, points of hip not discernable; withers, shoulders, and neck not obviously thin.	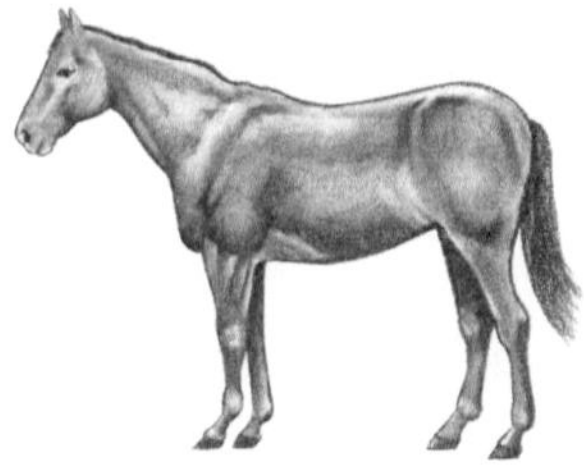
BCS 5	**Moderate:** Back is flat; ribs not visually distinguishable but easily felt; fat around tailhead beginning to feel spongy; withers appear rounded over spine; shoulders and neck blend smoothly into body.	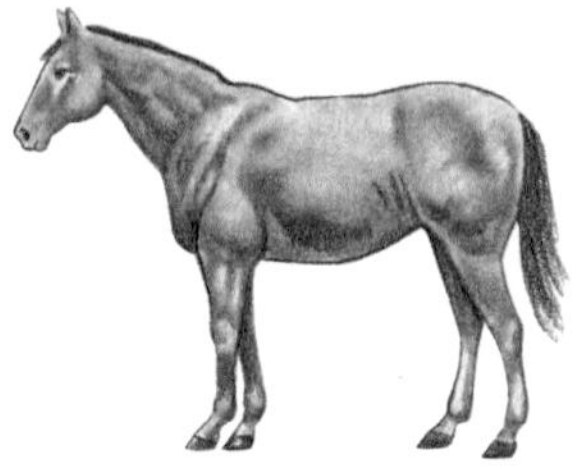
BCS 6	**Moderately fleshy:** May have slight crease down back; fat over ribs fleshy/spongy; fat around tailhead soft; fat beginning to be deposited along sides of the neck.	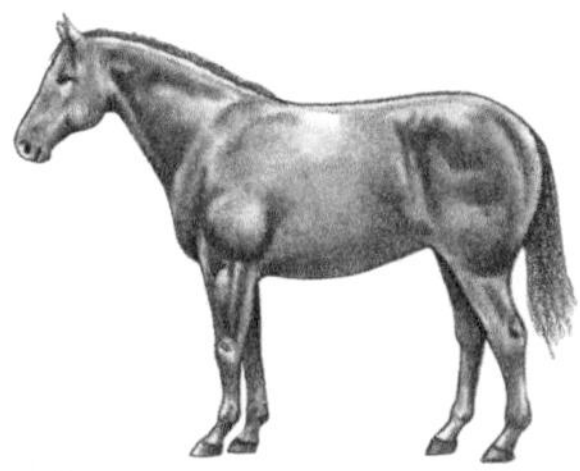
BCS 7	**Fleshy:** May have crease down back; individual ribs can be felt, but noticeable filling between ribs with fat; fat around tailhead soft; fat deposited along withers behind shoulders and along neck.	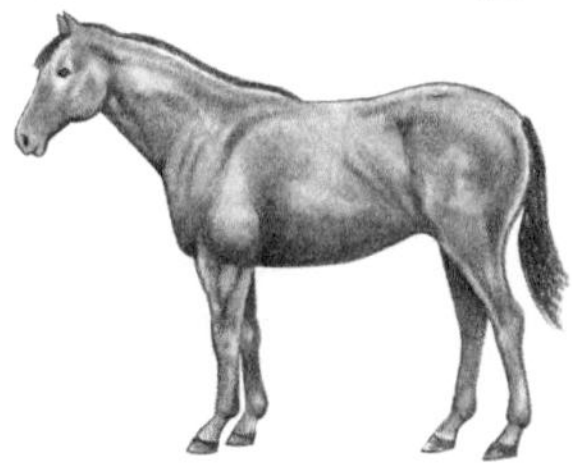
BCS 8	**Fat:** Crease down back; difficult to feel ribs; fat around tailhead very soft; area along withers filled with fat; area behind shoulders filled with fat; noticeable thickening of neck; fat deposited along inner thighs.	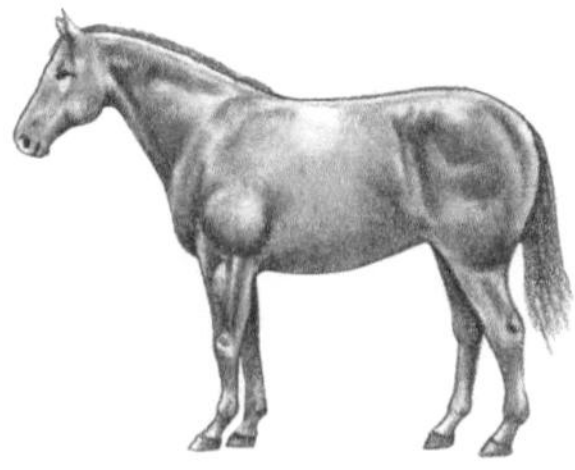
BCS 9	**Extremely fat:** Obvious crease down back; patchy fat appearing.	

Source: Henneke et al., 1983 (illustrations courtesy of Kentucky Equine Research www.ker.com)

Table 3.7 Workloads of horses in the light, moderate, heavy, and very heavy exercise categories for calculating DE requirements

Exercise category	*Description (based on weekly totals of work)*	*Types of events*	*DE requirements*
Light	1–3 hours per week; 40% walk, 50% trot, 10% canter.	Recreational riding, beginning of training programs, show horses (occasional).	DE (Mcal/d) = (0.0333 × BW) × 1.20
Moderate	3–5 hours per week; 30% walk, 55% trot, 10% canter, 5% low jumping, cutting, other skill work.	School horses, recreational riding, beginning of training/breaking, show horses (frequent), polo, ranch work.	DE (Mcal/d) = (0.0333 × BW) × 1.40
Heavy	4–5 hours per week; 20% walk, 50% trot, 15% canter, 15% gallop, jumping, other skill work.	Ranch work, polo, show horses (frequent, strenuous events). Low- to medium-level eventing. Race training (middle stages).	DE (Mcal/d) = (0.0333 × BW) × 1.60
Very heavy	Various; ranges from 1 hour per week speed work to 6–12 hours per week slow work.	Racing (quarter horse, thoroughbred, standardbred, endurance), elite three-day event.	DE (Mcal/d) = (0.0363 × BW) × 1.9

Source: NRC, 2007

In practice, the digestible energy (MJ/d) can be calculated using the formula: DE (MJ/d) = DE (Mcal) × 4.183.

Step 6: Calculate the forage requirement

Forage is a vital component of a horse's diet, providing essential fiber and nutrients and promoting healthy digestion.

- **General forage intake:** For horses at a healthy weight, provide forage ad libitum (free-choice) or a minimum of 1.5% of their body weight in DM per day. This means that a 500-kg horse should consume at least 7.5 kg of forage DM per day.

- **High-intensity work:** Horses in very high-intensity work may require a minimum of 1.25% of their body weight in forage DM per day (Harris et al., 2017).
- **Weight-loss program:** Horses undergoing a weight-loss program should be fed no less than 1% of their body weight in forage DM per day (Harris et al., 2017).

Adjust the amount based on the horse's individual needs and energy requirements. Consult with a veterinarian or equine nutritionist for specific guidance on managing weight loss in horses.

Understanding dry matter: When discussing forage intake, two terms are commonly used: as-fed basis and dry matter basis.

- **As-fed basis** refers to the amount of forage, including its water content, while DM refers to the nutrient value of the forage without water.
- **Dry matter** content varies among different forage types (e.g., hay, haylage, pasture), and it is important to know the DM percentage to calculate forage intake accurately.

Step 7: Choose forage types

To fully understand the value of a forage and its impact as part of the horse's diet, a laboratory nutrient analysis is recommended, and an estimation of the energy content should be made (Harris et al., 2017). This becomes particularly important when feeding horses with health disorders (e.g., low body condition score, obesity, laminitis, polysaccharide storage myopathy). The dry matter content of forage sources is a parameter that should be considered when calculating a diet for horses (Table 3.8). The hygienic quality of forages must be a key consideration, as poor hygienic quality can lead to reduced intakes or significant health problems. At a minimum, regular visual and olfactory inspections should be undertaken, and poor-quality forage should be appropriately disposed of.

Table 3.8 Typical DM content (%) of various forage types

Forage type	*Typical DM content (%)*
Hay	87–92
Haylage (dry)	50–80
Haylage (wet)	35–50
Silage	25–50
Lucerne (alfalfa)	88–92
Grass	15–35

Source: NRC, 2007; Geor et al., 2013

Benchmarks for microorganism contamination should be considered. Changes in forage should be done gradually to allow the hindgut microbiota to adapt, especially if the nutrient composition (energy, protein, WSC) is unknown or known to differ considerably due to changes in plant species, growth stage, and preservation technique. In such instances, an adaptation period of at least two and possibly more than three weeks may be required.

In this example, a healthy four-year-old thoroughbred mare with a body weight of 500 kg, good body condition score (BCS 5/9), and engaged in medium work, the calculation for the hay requirement can be outlined as follows:

- Once the horse's body weight is known, the estimation of the daily forage intake can begin.
- For a 500-kg horse, the minimum forage intake is calculated by multiplying the body weight by 1.5%, resulting in a minimum DM requirement of 7.5 kg of forage.
- To convert the dry matter amount to an as-fed basis, divide the DM value by the DM percentage of the hay. In this example, with a DM content of 90% for the hay, the calculation is as follows: 7.5 kg of forage DM / 90% DM of hay = 8.3 kg of hay as fed, which represents the minimum requirement for this horse.

If the mare were engaged in high-intensity work such as racing, the minimum DM forage requirement would be 1%–1.25% of her body weight, resulting in a minimum DM requirement of 5–6.25 kg. Converting this amount to an as-fed basis using the same hay DM percentage (90%) would yield a minimum requirement of 5.5–6.9 kg of hay per day.

Step 8: Calculate the appropriate forage-to-concentrate ratio in the diet and choose concentrate feed sources

The ideal forage-to-concentrate ratio can vary depending on factors such as the horse's age, weight, activity level, and specific nutritional requirements. However, a common recommendation is to provide a minimum of 50% to 70% of the diet as forage, with the remaining portion consisting of concentrates.

Adjustments may be necessary based on individual horse needs, health conditions, and other factors. Consulting with a veterinarian or equine nutritionist is recommended for personalized guidance and ensuring the horse's nutritional needs are being met.

If the forage intake falls below the minimum forage DM requirements for a horse, it is necessary to adjust the forage intake. Horses have specific dietary needs for fiber and maintaining digestive health, and inadequate forage intake can lead to issues such as digestive disturbances or an increased risk of colic.

The following adjustments can be made to ensure the horse receives sufficient forage:

- **Increase the quantity of forage:** Provide more hay, pasture, or other appropriate forage sources to meet or exceed the minimum forage DM requirement.
- **Evaluate the quality of forage:** Ensure that the forage being provided is of good quality and has adequate nutritional value. Poor-quality or low-nutrient forage may not meet the horse's dietary requirements even if the quantity is sufficient, as the horses won't eat enough of it.
- **Consider alternative forage sources:** If the current forage source is insufficient, explore other options, such as different types of hay, haylage, or alternative forage options to meet the horse's forage needs.

Step 9: Evaluate nutrient intake and balance the ration

Horse nutrient requirements are compared to horse intake for all nutrients, including energy, protein, fat, fiber, vitamins, and minerals. The diet is then adjusted to meet the horse's needs.

Water intake

Hydration management involves providing horses with continuous access to clean, fresh water and closely monitoring their water intake while ensuring the water sources are clean and free from contaminants. Elevated mineral content in water might result in decreased water consumption by horses. It's important to note that horses cannot drink from frozen water, and their intake may decrease if the water is excessively cold or hot.

Feeding schedule and management

- Divide the daily ration into multiple meals to promote proper digestion and prevent digestive issues. Aim for at least two to three feeds per day. It is often recommended not to provide more than 1–2 g starch/kg body weight per meal (Geor et al., 2007; Julliand et al., 2006), so dividing the starch intake into several meals is highly recommended.
- Maintain a consistent feeding schedule to establish a routine and minimize stress.
- Changes in forage should be made gradually, especially if the nutrient composition (energy, protein, WSC) is unknown or known to differ considerably due to changes in plant species, growth stage, and preservation technique. In such instances, an adaptation period of at least two and possibly more than three weeks may be required (Harris et al., 2017).

Computer-based diet evaluation and formulation for horses

Computer-based diet evaluation and formulation for horses refers to using specialized software programs and digital tools to assess and design optimal dietary plans for horses. These computer programs are specifically developed to aid horse owners, trainers, and equine nutritionists in creating well-balanced and tailored diets based on individual horse requirements.

The process typically involves inputting relevant information about the horse, such as age, breed, body weight, body condition, activity level, and any specific health conditions or dietary restrictions. The software then analyzes this data and generates comprehensive reports or recommendations for the horse's nutritional needs.

Some common features and functionalities of computer-based diet evaluation and formulation programs for horses may include:

- **Nutrient analysis:** The software has a library with the nutritional content of various feed ingredients and calculates the overall nutrient composition of the diet. It considers essential macronutrients (carbohydrates, proteins, and fats) and micronutrients (vitamins and minerals) to ensure proper balance.
- **Feeding recommendations:** Based on the input information, the software generates feeding recommendations and suggests appropriate quantities of different feed components to meet the horse's energy requirements and nutrient needs. This can include guidance on forage intake, concentrate feeds, supplements, and water requirements.
- **Nutritional analysis of forages and feeds:** Many programs incorporate databases with detailed nutritional profiles of commonly used forages, concentrates, and supplements. This enables accurate nutrient content assessment and helps in selecting appropriate feed options.
- **Monitoring and adjustments:** The software often allows users to track and monitor the horse's diet over time. Regular evaluations can be performed to assess the effectiveness of the current feeding plan and make necessary adjustments as per changing requirements or goals.
- **Research-based algorithms:** The software programs are developed based on scientific research and expertise in equine nutrition, ensuring that the calculations and recommendations align with current knowledge and best practices.

Popular computer-based diet evaluation and formulation programs for horses include PC-Horse and FRASC (Feed Ration Analysis and Suggestion Companion). These programs assist horse owners and professionals in creating and managing well-balanced diets, optimizing the horse's health, performance, and overall well-being.

These software programs offer convenience, accuracy, and time-saving benefits. They automate complex calculations, consider various nutrient requirements, and help balance the diet based on individual needs. By utilizing databases of nutritional profiles for forages, feeds, and supplements, the programs aid in selecting appropriate feed options.

However, it's essential to be aware of their limitations. The accuracy of recommendations relies on the accuracy and completeness of the input data, and individual variations may not be fully accounted for in estimating requirements. The quality and comprehensiveness of the feed ingredient database can impact the accuracy of nutrient calculations. Software programs should not replace the expertise of qualified equine nutritionists or veterinarians with equine nutrition expertise, who consider additional factors beyond nutrient requirements. These programs should be used in conjunction with professional advice and regular monitoring to ensure the best outcomes for equine nutrition.

References

Agar, C., Gemmill, R., Hollands, T., & Freeman, S. L. (2016). The use of nutritional supplements in dressage and eventing horses. *Veterinary Record Open*, *3*(1). https://doi.org/10.1136/vetreco-2015-000154

Burk, A. O., & Williams, C. A. (2008). Feeding management practices and supplement use in top-level event horses. *Comparative Exercise Physiology*, *5*(2), 85. https://doi.org/10.1017/S1478061508062786

Carroll, C. L., & Huntington, P. J. (1988). Body condition scoring and weight estimation of horses. *Equine Veterinary Journal*, *20*(1), 41–45. https://doi.org/10.1111/j.2042-3306.1988.tb01451.x

Copper, J. J., & Mason, G. J. (1998). The identification of abnormal behaviour and behavioural problems in stabled horses and their relationship to horse welfare: A comparative review. *Equine Veterinary Journal*, *30*(S27), 5–9. https://doi.org/10.1111/j.2042-3306.1998.tb05136.x

CVB Centraal Veevoeder Bureau (2005) CVB tabellenboek voeding paarden en pony's. *The new energy system for horses, Energie Waarde voor Paarden.*

Dosi, M. C. M., Kirton, R., Hallsworth, S., Keen, J. A., & Morgan, R. A. (2020). Inducing weight loss in native ponies: Is straw a viable alternative to hay? *Veterinary Record*, *187*(8). https://doi.org/10.1136/vr.105793

Drogoul, C., de Fombelle, A., & Julliand, V. (2001). Feeding and microbial disorders in horses: 2: Effect of three hay:grain ratios on digesta passage rate and digestibility in ponies. *Journal of Equine Veterinary Science*, *21*(10), 487–491. https://doi.org/10.1016/S0737-0806(01)70211-0

El Shorafa, W. M., Feaster, J. P., & Ott, E. A. (1979). Horse metacarpal bone: Age, ash content, cortical area and failure stress interrelationships. *Journal of Animal Science*, *49*(4), 979–982. https://doi.org/10.2527/jas1979.494979x

Garcia, E. I. C., Elghandour, M. M. M. Y., Khusro, A., Alcala-Canto, Y., Tirado-González, D. N., Barbabosa-Pliego, A., & Salem, A. Z. M. (2022). Dietary supplements of vitamins E, C, and β-Carotene to reduce oxidative stress in horses: An overview. *Journal of Equine Veterinary Science*, *110*, 103863. https://doi.org/10.1016/j.jevs.2022.103863

Geor, R., Harris, P., & Coenen, M. (2013). *Equine applied and clinical nutrition* (1st ed.). Elsevier Saunders, 66–68, 97, 414, 461.

Geor, R. J., & Harris, P. A. (2007). How to minimize gastrointestinal disease associated with carbohydrate nutrition in horses. *AAEP Proceeding*, *53*, 178–185.

Geor, R. J., Harris, P. A., & Green, E. M. (2007). *How to minimize gastrointestinal disease associated with carbohydrate nutrition in horses.* https://api.semanticscholar.org/CorpusID:43406636

Grimwood, K., Penaluna, L.-A., & Brown, H. (2016). A preliminary investigation into the mineral intake of horses in the UK. *Journal of Equine Veterinary Science*, *36*, 44–48. https://doi.org/10.1016/j.jevs.2015.09.012

Harris, P. A., Ellis, A. D., Fradinho, M. J., Jansson, A., Julliand, V., Luthersson, N., Santos, A. S., & Vervuert, I. (2017). Review: Feeding conserved forage to horses: Recent advances and recommendations. *Animal*, *11*(6), 958–967. https://doi.org/10.1017/S1751731116002469

Henneke, D. R., Potter, G. D., Kreider, J. L., & Yeates, B. F. (1983). Relationship between condition score, physical measurements and body fat percentage in mares. *Equine Veterinary Journal*, *15*(4), 371–372. https://doi.org/10.1111/j.2042-3306.1983.tb01826.x

Highfill, J. L., Potter, G. D., Eller, E. M., Gibbs, P. G., Scott, B. D., & Hood, D. M. (2005). Comparative absorption of calcium fed in varying chemical forms and effects on absorption of phosphorus and magnesium. *Proceedings 19th Equine Science Society*, 37–42.

Honoré, E. K., & Uhlinger, C. A. (1994). Equine feeding practices in central North Carolina: A preliminary survey. *Journal of Equine Veterinary Science*, *14*(8), 424–429. https://doi.org/10.1016/S0737-0806(06)82009-5

Hymøller, L., & Jensen, S. K. (2015). We know next to nothing about vitamin D in horses! *Journal of Equine Veterinary Science*, *35*(10), 785–792. https://doi.org/10.1016/j.jevs.2015.06.010

Ireland, J. L., Clegg, P. D., McGowan, C. M., McKane, S. A., & Pinchbeck, G. L. (2011). A cross-sectional study of geriatric horses in the United Kingdom. Part 1: Demographics and management practices. *Equine Veterinary Journal*, *43*(1), 30–36. https://doi.org/10.1111/j.2042-3306.2010.00145.x

Julliand, V., De Fombelle, A., & Varloud, M. (2006). Starch digestion in horses: The impact of feed processing. *Livestock Science*, *100*(1), 44–52. https://doi.org/10.1016/j.livprodsci.2005.11.001

Kaya-Karasu, G., Huntington, P. J., Iben, C., & Murray, J.-A. (2018). Feeding and management practices for racehorses in Turkey. *Journal of Equine Veterinary Science*, *61*, 108–113. https://doi.org/10.1016/j.jevs.2017.04.009

Kronfeld, D. S. (2001). Body fluids and exercise: Replacement strategies. *Journal of Equine Veterinary Science*, *21*(8), 368–375. https://doi.org/10.1016/S0737-0806(01)70003-2

Lawrence, L. A., Ott, E. A., Asquith, R. L., & Miller, G. J. (1987). Influence of dietary iron on growth, tissue mineral composition, apparent phosphorus absorption and chemical properties of bone. *Proc. 10th Equine Nutr. Physiol. Soc. Symp*, *10*, 563–572.

Lindinger, M. I. (2022). Oral electrolyte and water supplementation in horses. *Veterinary Sciences*, *9*(11), 626. https://doi.org/10.3390/vetsci9110626

Lindinger, M. I., & Cairns, S. P. (2021). Regulation of muscle potassium: Exercise performance, fatigue and health implications. *European Journal of Applied Physiology*, *121*(3), 721–748. https://doi.org/10.1007/s00421-020-04546-8

Medina, B., Girard, I. D., Jacotot, E., & Julliand, V. (2002). Effect of a preparation of Saccharomyces cerevisiae on microbial profiles and fermentation patterns in the large intestine of horses fed a high fiber or a high starch diet. *Journal of Animal Science*, *80*(10), 2600. https://doi.org/10.2527/2002.80102600x

NRC. (2007). *Nutrient requirements of horses* (6th ed.). National Academies Press. https://doi.org/10.17226/11653

Pagan, J. D. 2001. Factors affecting mineral digestibility. In: J. D. Pagan and R. J. Geor (Ed.) *Advances in Equine Nutrition II*. pp. 13–27. Nottingham University Press. Nottingham, United Kingdom.

Regulation. (2009). Regulation (EC) No 767/2009 of the European Parliament and of the Council of 13 July 2009 on the placing on the market and use of feed. *Amending European Parliament and Council*.

Richards, N., Hinch, G., & Rowe, J. (2006). The effect of current grain feeding practices on hindgut starch fermentation and acidosis in the Australian racing Thoroughbred. *Australian Veterinary Journal*, *84*(11), 402–407. https://doi.org/10.1111/j.1751-0813.2006.00059.x

Vervuert, I., Voigt, K., Hollands, T., Cuddeford, D., & Coenen, M. (2009). Effect of feeding increasing quantities of starch on glycaemic and insulinaemic responses in healthy horses. *The Veterinary Journal*, *182*(1), 67–72. https://doi.org/10.1016/j.tvjl.2008.04.011

CHAPTER 4

Nutrition-related health disorders in horses

Nutrition plays a crucial role in the overall health and well-being of horses. Imbalances or deficiencies in their diet can lead to various nutrition-related health disorders. Several nutrition-related health disorders can affect horses.

4.1 The role of nutrition in developmental orthopedic diseases in horses

DOD stands for developmental orthopedic disease, which refers to a group of skeletal disorders that affect young, growing horses (Figure 4.1). These conditions primarily occur during the development and maturation of the skeletal system, typically in horses up to three years of age. DOD encompasses various conditions that affect different parts of the musculoskeletal system, including bones, joints, cartilage, and ligaments.

Some common types of DOD in horses include:

- **Osteochondritis dissecans (OCD):** OCD is characterized by the presence of cartilage defects or fragments within a joint. It principally affects the hock, fetlock, and stifle and shoulder joints.
- **Epiphysitis:** Also known as physitis, epiphysitis involves the enlargement of the growth plates of certain long bones in young horses. It can result in abnormal bone growth and deformities, typically seen in the lower cannon bone of both limbs in foals and weanlings or above the knee in yearlings.
- **Angular limb deformities:** Angular limb deformities refer to abnormal angular deviations in the alignment of a limb. This can occur due to unequal growth rates of the bones on either side of a joint, leading to

DOI: 10.1201/9781003379355-4

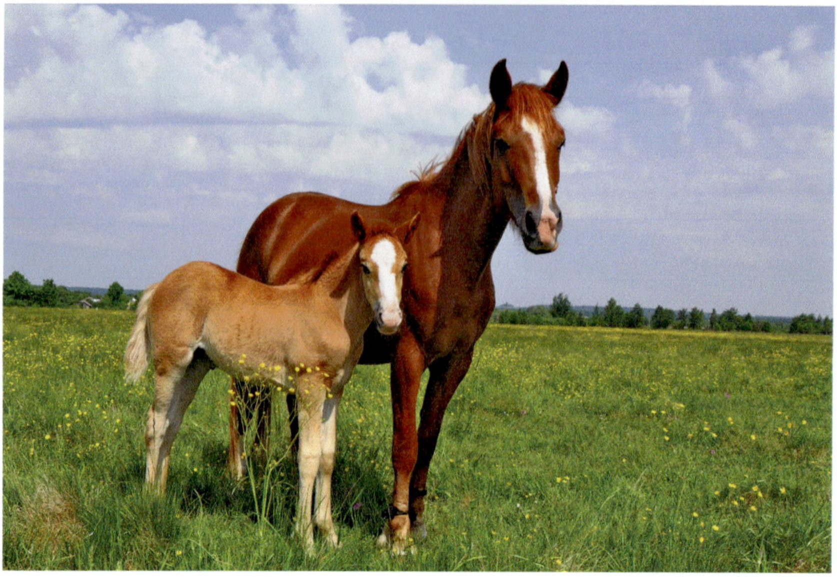

Figure 4.1 A healthy foal with legs free of developmental orthopedic diseases.

issues such as valgus (outward deviation) or varus (inward deviation) deformities.

- **Flexural deformities:** Flexural deformities involve abnormal or excessive contraction of tendons and ligaments, leading to problems with limb extension or flexion. This can result in conditions such as contracted tendons or clubfoot.
- **Wobblers:** Wobblers may be caused by spinal abnormalities, infection, or injury. Horses with wobbler syndrome frequently exhibit uncoordinated gaits.
- **Subchondral bone cysts:** Subchondral bone cysts typically form during the development of the foal's skeletal system. Subchondral cystic lesions are most commonly found in the medial femoral condyle of the stifle. The two most common reasons are failure of proper ossification in foals and subchondral bone trauma.

The exact causes of DOD in horses are multifactorial, and risk factors can include genetic predisposition, nutritional imbalances, rapid growth, big newborn foals, conformational abnormalities, trauma, exercise, environment, and management practices. Proper nutrition, appropriate exercise, balanced growth, and regular veterinary care are crucial in preventing and managing DOD in young horses.

Proper nutrition is crucial in reducing the risk of DOD in horses. Some dietary recommendations to help reduce the risk of DOD (Ahmadi et al., 2021; Kronfeld et al., 1990; Lepeule et al., 2009; Pagan, 2003) are:

- **Balanced diet:** Ensure that your horse's diet provides a balanced ratio of essential nutrients, including protein, energy, minerals (such as calcium and phosphorus), trace minerals (like copper and zinc), and vitamins. Pregnancy is a vital time in terms of dietary balance related to DOD.
- **Energy intake:** Avoid overfeeding pregnant mares and young horses, as large foals, excessive weight gain, and rapid growth can increase the risk of DOD. Monitor their body condition regularly and adjust their feed intake accordingly. Avoid excessive concentrate or high-starch diets, as they can contribute to rapid growth and increase the risk of DOD.
- **Avoid excessive grain/starch feeding:** Limit the intake of concentrates or grain-based feeds in young horses and late pregnant mares. Concentrates should be fed in moderation and should not be the primary component of the diet. Excessive intake of sugars and starches can lead to rapid growth and an increased risk of DOD.
- **Access to lush pasture:** If your horse has access to pasture, manage grazing time and ensure that the pasture is not overly lush or high in non-structural carbohydrates. Excessive intake of sugars and starches from rich pasture can lead to rapid growth and an increased risk of DOD. Mares and young horses on lush pasture usually need a low-intake (and low-energy) balancer pellet rather than a full feed.
- **Mineral balance:** Ensure that the diet contains appropriate levels and ratios of minerals, especially calcium, phosphorus, copper, and zinc. These minerals are critical for proper bone development.
- **Feeding schedule:** Establish a consistent feeding routine with regular meal times and small meals. Avoid prolonged periods of fasting or irregular feeding schedules, as they can disrupt proper growth and digestion. Unregulated group feeding may allow excessive feed intake by dominant horses.

4.2 The role of nutrition in colic

Colic is a common digestive disorder of horses. It is not a disease but a generic form of abdominal pain. The signs of colic can vary depending on the severity and underlying cause, but they may include frequent pawing or kicking at the abdomen, rolling or attempting to roll, restlessness or agitation, loss of appetite or decreased feed intake, absence or reduction of bowel movements, increased heart rate and respiratory rate, sweating or cold extremities, and stretching out as if to urinate without producing urine (Figure 4.2).

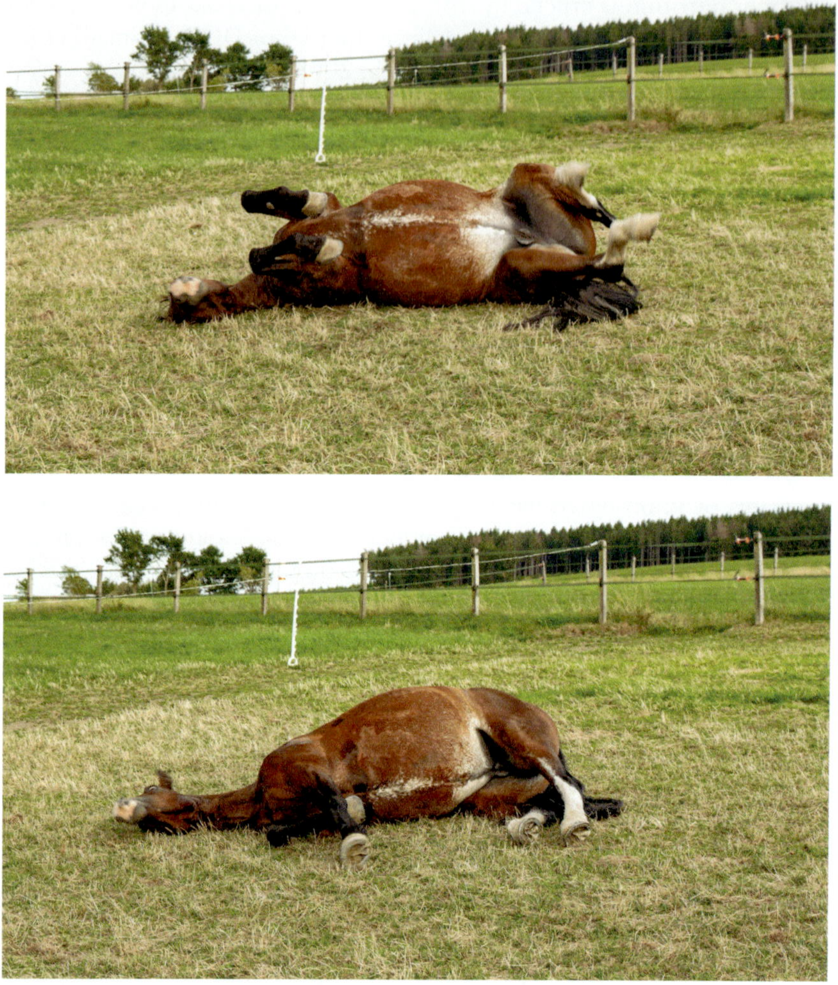

Figure 4.2 The colic horse is in pain.

Colic is the most common emergency condition and a significant cause of death in horses (Bowden et al., 2020; Cohen et al., 1999; Traub-Dargatz et al., 2001). Colic occurs more frequently in horses that have previously experienced it. A study of 127 horses with a veterinary-diagnosed episode of colic found an incidence of 50 episodes per 100 horse-years (Scantlebury et al., 2015). The overall mortality rate for colic was 0.45 deaths per 100 horse-years in thoroughbred training premises in the UK (Hillyer et al., 2001). The proportional mortality rate of colic, 28%, was higher than for any other cause of death (Tinker et al., 1997b). Colic can range from mild and self-limiting cases to severe and life-threatening conditions. Colic may occur due to different causes, including nutrition and feeding management

(Durham, 2009). In horses, most of these problems involve the gastrointestinal tract, but diseases of other structures within or associated with the abdomen, such as the kidneys, liver, uterus, bladder, peritoneum, or spleen, may also result in signs of colic (Traub-Dargatz et al., 2001). Every horse group has unique intrinsic or extrinsic characteristics related to diet, management, or weather conditions, which may influence the occurrence of colic (Kaya et al., 2009) (Table 4.1).

The most frequently encountered types of colic in horses are:

- **Gas colic:** This type of colic is caused by an excessive accumulation of gas in the horse's gastrointestinal tract. Gas colic can be caused by rapid changes in diet, ingestion of spoiled food, or the fermentation of certain feeds. It often presents as mild to moderate discomfort. However, gas can also contribute to displacements and other surgical colic.
- **Impaction colic:** Impaction colic occurs when there is a blockage or obstruction in the horse's digestive system, commonly in the large colon or small colon. It is often caused by inadequate water intake, poor-quality forage, ingesting sand or foreign objects, or insufficient exercise. Impaction colic can range from mild to severe discomfort.
- **Spasmodic colic:** This type of colic is characterized by intermittent spasms or contractions of the horse's intestinal muscles, leading to pain and discomfort. The exact cause is not always clear, but it can be related to changes in diet, stress, or improper feeding practices.
- **Displacement or twisted gut colic:** This is a more severe and potentially life-threatening type of colic. It occurs when a portion of the horse's intestine becomes twisted or displaced, leading to an obstruction and compromising blood flow. This can result in severe pain and rapid deterioration, and surgical intervention is usually necessary to correct the twist or displacement.

Enteritis or colitis: Enteritis refers to inflammation of the small intestine, while colitis refers to inflammation of the large intestine. Both conditions can cause colic symptoms in horses. They are often caused by bacterial or viral infections, parasites, or dietary factors. The majority of equine colic cases are classified as "spasmodic," "gas," or "non-specific" (Archer & Proudman, 2006). Treatment for colic depends on the underlying cause and may involve medical management or surgical intervention in severe cases. Colic is a veterinary emergency, and prompt diagnosis and treatment are crucial. Horse owners should contact a veterinarian immediately if they suspect their horse is experiencing colic symptoms.

Prevention of colic involves proper feeding practices, regular dental care, parasite control, and maintaining a consistent exercise routine for the horse.

Table 4.1 The most common causes of colic in horses

Possible feeding and management risk factors	*(Cohen et al., 1995)*	*(Reeves et al., 1996)*	*(Kaneene et al., 1997)*	*(Tinker et al., 1997b)*	*(Cohen et al., 1999)*	*(Hudson et al., 2001)*	*(Scantlebury et al., 2015)*	*(Hillyer et al., 2001)*	*(Kaya et al., 2009)*
Study location	US	US	US	US	US	US	UK	UK	Austria
Study duration	15 months	10 months	2 years	1 year	1 year	13 months	4 months	1 year	1 year
Number of horses	1642	842	3925	948	2060	364	127	80	2743
Recent change of diet	#				#		#	#	0
Recent change of concentrate				#		#		#	0
Recent change of hay					#	#		#	0
High amount of concentrate		#		#		#			#
Inadequate intake of water	#	#	#						#
Recent change of exercise	#								0
Recent change of stabling	#			0	#			#	0

Recent change means two weeks prior to examination; # = increased risk of colic, 0 = no association.

In general, good nutritional and feeding management might reduce colic risk:

- **Consistent feeding routine:** Establish a regular feeding schedule and stick to it as much as possible. Horses thrive on routine, and sudden changes in feeding times or amounts can disrupt their digestive system and increase the risk of colic. Feed meals at the same times each day, with a consistent interval between meals.
- **Small meals:** Providing small, frequent meals also prevents colic in horses, promoting efficient digestion in the gastrointestinal tract (GIT).
- **High-quality forage:** Provide horses with good-quality forage, such as hay or pasture, as the primary component of their diet. High-fiber forage helps maintain proper gut motility and reduces the risk of impaction colic. Ensure the forage is free from mold, dust, or contaminants that could harm the horse's digestive system (Kaya et al., 2009). A recent decrease in pasture availability has been associated with increased colic risk (Hudson et al., 2001).
- **Adequate hay supply and lower-concentrate intakes:** The minimal amount of roughage recommended to maintain the optimal functioning of hindgut microbes is equivalent to 2% (84% to 90% dry matter) per kg BW per day (Coenen et al., 2011). One approach to mitigate potential adverse effects involves altering the sequence of distributing concentrate and hay. Specifically, compared to feeding concentrate before hay, distributing hay first has been observed to reduce alterations in the hindgut physicochemical environment, which could otherwise disrupt the microbial ecosystems in the hindgut (Jensen et al., 2012; Philippeau et al., 2009). Providing high levels of concentrate, exceeding 2.5 kg/day of dry matter, elevates the likelihood of colic compared to not feeding concentrate at all (Tinker et al., 1997a). Consequently, reducing the amount of concentrate in the feed lowers the associated risk of colic, although low starch concentrates will have lower risks than traditional grains.
- **Adequate water supply:** Ensure horses have access to clean, fresh water at all times. Proper hydration is crucial for maintaining normal digestive function and preventing impactions. In colder weather, use heated water sources to prevent water from freezing.
- **Pasture turnout:** Daily turnout for >12 hours helps promote normal gastrointestinal motility and prevent stagnation in the digestive system.
- **Gradual diet changes:** Introduce dietary changes gradually to allow the horse's digestive system and microbiome to adjust. Abrupt changes in feed type or quantity can upset the microbial balance in the gut and lead to digestive disturbances. Make any dietary adjustments over several days to several weeks, gradually replacing old feed with new feed.
- **Feed management:** Avoid feeding horses on the ground, as they may ingest sand, dirt, or other foreign objects that can contribute to colic.

However, using ground-level feed bins allows horses to eat with their head down and encourages drainage of any respiratory secretions. Use elevated feeders or mangers to minimize the risk of ingestion of contaminants. Additionally, use slow-feeders or haynets with smaller openings to promote slower consumption and reduce the risk of over-eating or bolting food.

4.3 The role of nutrition in equine gastric ulcer syndrome (EGUS)

Gastric ulcers, also known as equine gastric ulcer syndrome, are a very common digestive disorder affecting horses' stomach lining. The past 20 years have seen rapid developments in the diagnosis, treatment, and research of EGUS. However, there are still many misunderstandings about EGUS among horse owners, as suggested by a review of social media and equine websites (Marlin et al., 2019).

Horses have the potential to develop stomach ulcers in two areas: the upper (squamous) regions of the stomach are affected by Equine Squamous Gastric Disease (ESGD), while the lower (glandular) are affected by Equine Glandular Gastric Disease (EGGD) (Figure 4.3). The prevalence of ESGD varies depending on the group sampled and the exercise level or program. The prevalence of ESGD at post-mortem has been described as 61% in feral

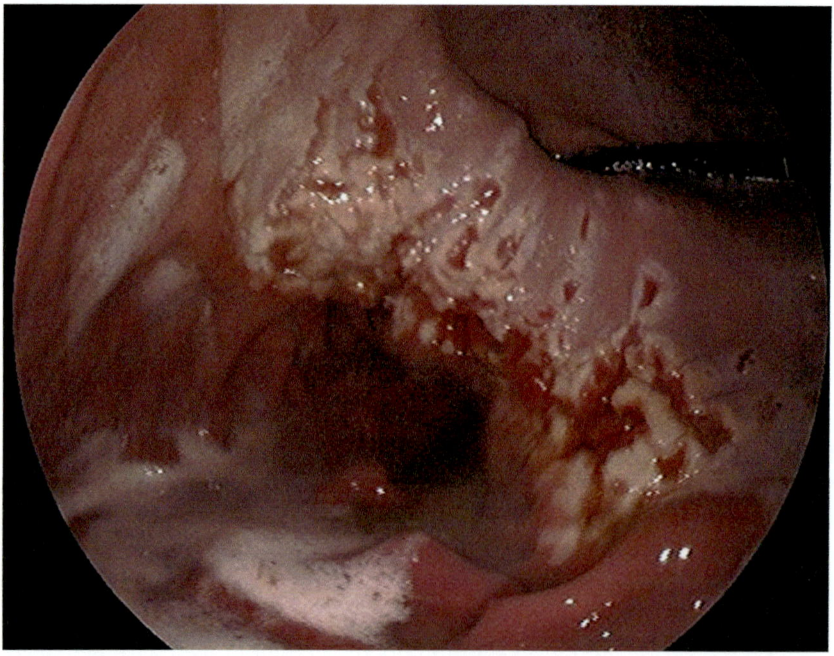

Figure 4.3 Multiple severe ulcers in the stomach regions.

horses in the UK (Ward et al., 2015) and 64% in equids in a safari park (Lamglait et al., 2017). In the UK, a survey conducted in abattoirs revealed a prevalence of EGGD at 71% in domesticated horses, whereas the prevalence was 30% in feral horses (Ward et al., 2015). Even when their stomach is empty, horses produce hydrochloric acid at varying rates, increasing the likelihood of gastric ulceration, particularly in the squamous area, which has no protection against acid. In contrast, the glandular region has several protective mechanisms against acid damage.

Continuous acid secretion occurs in horses' stomachs, and when horses have access to hay, their gastric acidity is considerably lower compared to horses that have fasted for 24 hours. While it may appear that feeding would increase gastric acid secretion, the buffering capacity of the feed and the high levels of bicarbonate present in equine saliva seem to neutralize gastric acid. Horses only produce saliva when the stretch receptors of the mouth are activated by chewing or stimulation (Smyth et al., 1998). EGUS is classified into various grades, depending on the severity and extent of the ulcers identified:

Grade 1: The stomach lining remains intact, but there are regions of reddening.

Grade 2: The stomach exhibits small, single, or multiple ulcers.

Grade 3: The stomach features large, single, or multiple ulcers.

Grade 4: The stomach has extensive ulcers, often merging to create areas of deep ulceration.

Risk factors of EGUS

- **Dietary factors:** Prolonged periods without food, intermittent feeding, and high-starch diets (grains, sweet feeds) are common contributors to gastric ulcers in horses. These feeding practices can disrupt the natural buffering mechanisms of the stomach and increase the risk of ulcers. The consumption of grain-based or high-starch meals, coupled with extended periods of fasting, results in excessive gastric acid production without sufficient saliva for buffering the acid. Furthermore, the fermentation of starch in the stomach produces volatile fatty acids (VFAs), which can damage the squamous epithelium of the stomach (Sorrentino et al., 2019). The likelihood of squamous ulcers rises when straw is the only forage option, when starch intake exceeds 1 g/kg body weight per meal, when water is not accessible in the turnout paddock, and when the time gap between forage feedings exceeds 6 hours (Luthersson et al., 2009).

- **Stress:** Intense exercise, training, competition, transportation, or changes in the horse's environment or routine can create stress, which may increase the likelihood of gastric ulcers.
- **Exercise level:** Horses engaged in intense training or high levels of physical activity are more likely to develop EGUS than those with less strenuous exercise routines. Exercising ≥5 days per week, racing below expectation, and training are risk factors for EGGD in thoroughbred racehorses (Sykes et al., 2019), although EGGD tends to be more a disease of warmblood performance horses. Risk factors specific to ESGD include an increased time in work, current training (Dionne et al., 2003), or recent racing (Jonsson & Egenvall, 2010). The exact mechanisms underlying this association are not fully understood, but several factors have been suggested. Intense exercise can increase gastric acid production and reduce blood flow to the stomach, which may contribute to the development of ulcers. Trotting has been shown to contribute to the splashing of acid stomach contents, which can then damage the squamous mucosa, leading to ESGD. Additionally, the physical movement and jarring effects during exercise can disrupt the protective mucus layer in the stomach, making the glandular gastric mucosa more susceptible to damage from acid. A recent study examined the prevalence and severity of EGUS in a group of 28 riding horses with varying levels of physical activity and training intensity (Stefanyk & Slivinska, 2021). The study included two horse breeds. In the period of intermediate training, the prevalence of EGUS increased from 10% to 46%, with varying degrees of mucosal defects. The results demonstrated a significant correlation between training intensity and gastric ulceration.
- **Medications:** Some medications, such as non-steroidal anti-inflammatory drugs (NSAIDs), can contribute to the development of gastric ulcers in horses.

Squamous and glandular ulcers have different risk factors, and diagnosis of each disease can only be made by gastroscopy. As previously stated, several risk factors play a role in the development of EGUS, and understanding these risk factors may help prevent EGUS (Table 4.2).

Symptoms of EGUS: The signs of gastric ulcers in horses can vary, with some horses not exhibiting any symptoms. Common signs include poor appetite, weight loss, behavioral changes (such as depression, aggression, or anxiety), poor body condition, dull coat, and intermittent colic or abdominal discomfort (Bezděková et al., 2008; DUKTI et al., 2010; Gough et al., 2020; Nieto et al., 2009). Some horses may only show poor athletic performance or aversion to training. However, there is limited scientific evidence to support this. Only a few studies have found a significant association between gastric ulcers and decreased performance (Franklin et al., 2008;

Table 4.2 The most common risk and protective factors for EGUS

Risk factors for EGUS	*Protective factors for EGUS*
Diets high in starch or concentrates, which are abundant in grains, can elevate gastric acid production and reduce saliva production. This condition increases the likelihood of developing ulcers.	Saliva secretion is an important part of the protective mechanism because saliva acts as a natural buffer for gastric acid, neutralizing it and protecting the stomach lining.
Irregular feeding patterns or prolonged fasting periods can result in increased gastric acid production due to the lack of the buffering effect of continuous saliva and feed intake. This makes the stomach lining more susceptible to damage.	Mucus secretion is a key aspect of EGUS protection because the stomach lining produces mucus that forms a protective layer, preventing direct contact between gastric acid and epithelial cells.
Physical stress factors such as intense exercise, training, travel, or competition can contribute to the development of gastric ulcers in horses. These stressors can disrupt normal gastric motility and increase the production of gastric acid.	Horses that have continuous access to forage or pasture have a lower incidence of gastric ulcers. Because regular fiber consumption stimulates saliva production and reduces stomach lining exposure to gastric acid, a fiber ball in the stomach reduces acid splash during exercise.
Management factors such as confinement in stables, limited turnout time, and lack of access to forage or pasture can contribute to stress and increase the risk of gastric ulcers.	Omega-6 fatty acids have been shown to increase the secretion of protective prostaglandins and reduce acid secretion, and long-chain omega-3 fatty acids have an anti-inflammatory effect, which is beneficial in EGGD cases.
NSAIDs increase the risk of gastric ulcers.	

Jonsson & Egenvall, 2010; Kaya-Karasu et al., 2016; Lo Feudo et al., 2022; Sykes et al., 2019). The high prevalence of EGUS in performance horses is likely iatrogenic, resulting from factors such as feeding management, confinement in stables, and exercise.

Treatment of EGUS: Treatment procedures usually consist of a combination of medication and management changes. Proton pump inhibitors (PPIs) or histamine receptor antagonists (H2 blockers) are commonly used to reduce acid production in the stomach and promote ulcer healing. Reducing stressors and following routine management practices may help in the healing process for gastric ulcers. Treatment procedures need to involve dietary changes. The act of mastication, which produces saliva, can potentially reduce the occurrence of gastric ulcers. This is because saliva acts as a buffer for gastric acid, helping to neutralize it. Additionally, saliva provides extra mucus that aids in protecting the gastric epithelium from damage. Long-stem (7.62 cm chop length) chaff-type forage mixed with grain may provide a way to increase salivation through increased mastication (Sorrentino et al., 2019). Providing alfalfa pellets in the diet can potentially decrease the occurrence and severity of EGGD (Julliand et al., 2023). This is likely attributed to the lower starch content and the elevated calcium content in alfalfa, which imparts a greater buffering capacity than other commonly used feeds. A lower prevalence and severity of gastric ulcers occur in horses kept on pasture with continuous feed availability than in horses stabled and fed with high-grain diets. As higher starch intakes are a risk factor, the diet should contain increased amounts of alternative energy sources such as fat and super fibers. In addition, oil has been shown to have physiological benefits, with corn oil (high omega-6) being shown to increase levels of protective prostaglandins and reduce acid secretion (Cargile et al., 2004). A recent study using a blend of long-chain omega-3 and omega-6 fatty acids resulted in a significant reduction in ESGD severity (Pagan et al., 2022). Therefore, it is recommended to:

- Provide free-choice access to good-quality forage, alfalfa, or pasture.
- Feed hay before exercise so there is a fiber ball in the stomach to reduce acid splash.
- Feed smaller, more frequent meals rather than large concentrate meals.
- Reduce starch intake.
- Increase fat intake to supply alternative energy sources. Long-chain omega-3 fatty acids from fish oil have an anti-inflammatory effect, so they would be beneficial for EGGD treatment, and a long-chain omega-3/6 blend has been shown to reduce the severity of ESGD.
- Minimize stress and maintain a consistent environment and routine.
- Consider using preventive medications under veterinary guidance during periods of increased stress or when necessary.
- Other dietary supplements, such as sucralfate, increase the success rate of treatment for EGGD cases (Sykes et al., 2015). Sucralfate is a complex salt that adheres to the glandular mucosa. Limited alternatives to oral omeprazole therapy have been investigated, including injectable forms, with sparsely published efficacy data available. The three best-studied alternatives include a prostaglandin E analog, another PPI, and drugs belonging to the H2 receptor antagonist class, such as ranitidine (Vokes et al., 2023).

4.4 The role of nutrition in obesity

Obesity in horses is a common health concern that can have serious consequences for their well-being.

In the body condition scoring (BCS) system for horses, a BCS of 9 is considered "extremely fat" or "obese" (Chapter 3, Tables 3.5 and 3.6). At this level, the horse has a large amount of body fat. Ribs and other bony structures are completely buried beneath a thick layer of fat (Figure 4.4). The spine and hip bones are not visible or palpable due to the excess fat deposits. The horse may have fat pads in multiple areas of the body, including the neck, shoulder, withers, tailhead, and behind the shoulders. The neck's crest is extremely thick and may droop to one side, filled with internal fat. Recognizing that some animals carry excessive fat in different regions of their body, Carter et al. also described the 0–5 cresty neck score (2009a). Recent research has shown that 21% and 19% of horses in the UK (Harker et al., 2011) and New York (Brooks et al., 2010), respectively, were considered "fleshy" with a BCS of >7. Obesity in horses can lead to various health problems, such as metabolic disease, laminitis, inflammation, cardiovascular changes, and/or arthritis (Pratt-Phillips & Munjizun, 2023). Obesity also negatively impacts exercise performance because of a combined inflammatory response, as well as the effects of excessive weight carriage on work effort and limb health (Pratt-Phillips & Munjizun, 2023).

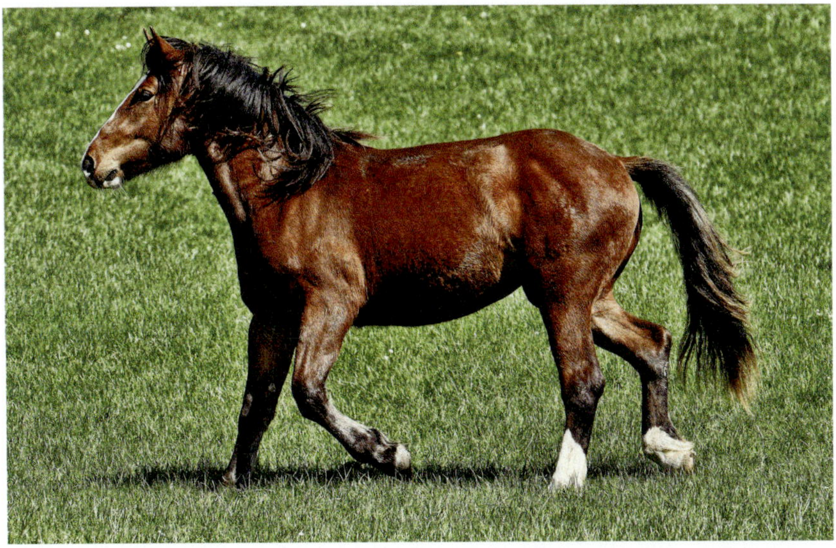

Figure 4.4 An illustration of an overweight horse with a BCS of 7 out of 9.

Causes

- **Breed predisposition:** Certain breeds have a higher susceptibility to obesity. The prevalence of equine obesity is observed across different regions, such as 24% in mature Icelandic horses in Denmark (Jensen et al., 2016) and up to 54% in leisure horses of diverse breeds in the UK (Stephenson et al., 2011), reaching 60% in Finnish horses (Karikoski et al., 2011). Obesity prevalence varies between horses and ponies. Obesity was three times more prevalent in pony breeds (31%) than in horses (10%), with a prevalence of 72% in the Shetland pony breed in Australia (Potter et al., 2016). Native cobs have a 14-fold higher prevalence of obesity, and native ponies appear to be at twice the risk of obesity as lightweight breeds in the Northern UK (Giles et al., 2014).
- **Overfeeding:** Obesity is caused primarily by an energy imbalance, in which energy from the diet exceeds energy expenditure. Providing horses with excessive amounts of high-calorie feeds, such as lush pasture, haylages, legume forages, and concentrates, can lead to obesity (D'Eath et al., 2009).
- **Grazing on rich pastures:** Horses with unrestricted access to lush pastures may consume more grass than they require, leading to weight gain. Previous research indicates that ponies can eat up to 4.9% of their body weight in dry matter (Longland et al., 2011) over 24 hours and up to 1% of their body weight (Ireland et al., 2012) when out at pasture for only 3 hours, indicating that some individuals can ingest significant amounts of grass, in even a short period out at pasture.
- **Lack of exercise:** Insufficient physical activity or confinement in small areas limits the horse's ability to burn calories and maintain a healthy weight.

Prevention and management

A balanced diet, controlled grazing, regular exercise, weight control, and veterinary guidance are crucial in addressing and managing obesity in horses.

- **Balanced diet:** Provide horses with a well-balanced diet that meets their nutritional requirements without excess calories. Straw may, accordingly, be an effective component of a weight loss management program (Jansson et al., 2021). It was recently suggested that horses should be fed at least 1.5% of BW on a dry matter (DM) basis of forage per day in order to support natural behavior and gut health (Harris et al., 2017). However, for some horses, even this amount of grass or legume forage may exceed energy requirements, especially during a weight loss program, and therefore, replacing part of the forage ration with low-energy straw could be a good alternative. A high-energy, forage-only diet alters the metabolic response to exercise and appears to have positive rather than negative effects on performance, with the exception of decreased glycogen stores (Jansson & Lindberg, 2012). Nonetheless, a forage-only diet will have mineral and vitamin deficiencies, necessitating the use of a low-intake feed balancer pellet to compensate.

- **Controlled grazing:** Monitor the amount of time and access horses have to pastures with rich grass. In an attempt to reduce horse body condition, owners have sought to restrict forage intake through a number of methods, including eliminating or decreasing the amount of time on pasture; however, restricted grazing is not always effective. Glunk et al. (2013) found that horses were able to increase their DM intake rates with restricted grazing time. Many horse owners are in need of management strategies that restrict pasture intake while maintaining a horse's natural environment (Glunk et al., 2013). Use grazing muzzles or strip-grazing techniques to limit their intake. The use of a grazing muzzle appears to offer a simple, affordable, and effective management strategy for restricting forage intakes of grazing horses, and it was found that using a grazing muzzle reduced forage intake by 83% when ponies grazed an autumn pasture with a sward height of 8–15 cm (Longland et al., 2011) (Figure 4.5).
- **Regular exercise:** To burn calories and maintain a healthy weight, make sure horses get regular exercise and physical activity. Exercise programs should be customized to the horse's age, performance level, and any underlying health issues such as laminitis. Swimming exercise has been shown to reduce insulin dysregulation in horses with hoof pain from laminitis.
- **Weight monitoring:** Monitor and record your horse's BCS regularly to track their weight and make necessary changes to their diet and

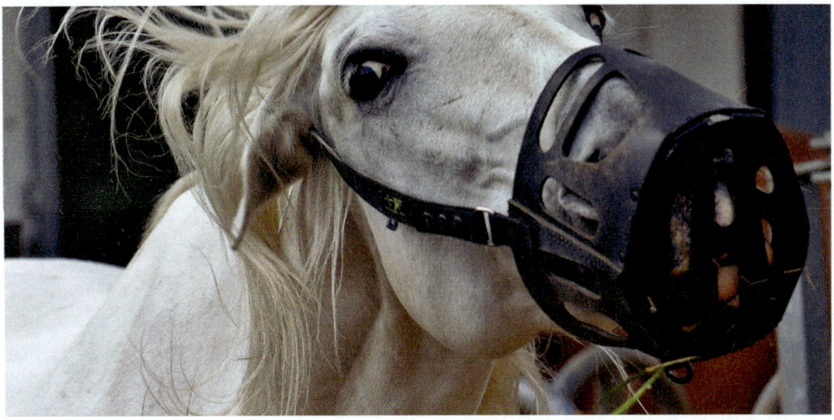

Figure 4.5 Image of a horse with a grazing muzzle.

exercise regimen. Neck circumference and cresty neck score are also important parameters in some obese horses.

4.5 The role of nutrition in laminitis

Laminitis is a severe and painful condition that affects horses' hooves and can cause lameness. It occurs when there is inflammation and damage to the sensitive laminae, which are the structures that connect the hoof wall to the pedal or coffin bone inside the hoof, potentially leading to the rotation of the bone (Figure 4.6). Laminitis can be a life-threatening condition if not managed properly. Laminitis remains an important condition in horses and ponies, not just because of the seriousness of the clinical signs and systemic changes involved but because of the potentially poor prognosis and increased likelihood of disease recurrence. Normal horses, exposed to sudden increases in grain consumption and concentrate, experience changes in cecal volume (increase), internal environment (lower pH), and the resident bacterial populations (higher total densities and different proportions of the various groups) (Goodson et al., 1988). There is increased fermentation in the small intestinal lumen when concentrate diets are fed. This is believed to induce increased intestinal permeability and associated endotoxemia in carbohydrate-induced laminitis (Weiss et al., 2000). Evidence from ponies and overweight, insulin-insensitive horses further demonstrates the importance of carbohydrate intake and digestion in the pathogenesis of laminitis (Field & Jeffcott, 1989).

The four experimental models are commonly used to investigate the pathogenesis of laminitis. The description of each model is as follows (Eades, 2017):

- **Carbohydrate overload (high starch):** This model involves feeding horses or ponies a large amount of carbohydrate-rich feed, such as grains or concentrates. The overload of starch in the digestive system can disrupt the microbial balance and lead to the production of lactic acid and other by-products, causing metabolic disturbances that can trigger laminitis (Figure 4.7).
- **Black walnut extract administration:** Black walnut shavings or extracts contain compounds known as juglone and related toxins, which can cause laminitis when horses come into contact with or ingest them. This model is used to study the toxic effects of juglone on the hoof laminae and its role in laminitis development.
- **Oligofructose (fructan) overload:** Fructans are complex sugars found in certain grasses, such as cool-season grasses. In an experimental model, horses or ponies are fed a large amount of fructan-rich forage or grass, which can ferment in the hindgut and produce by-products that can trigger laminitis.

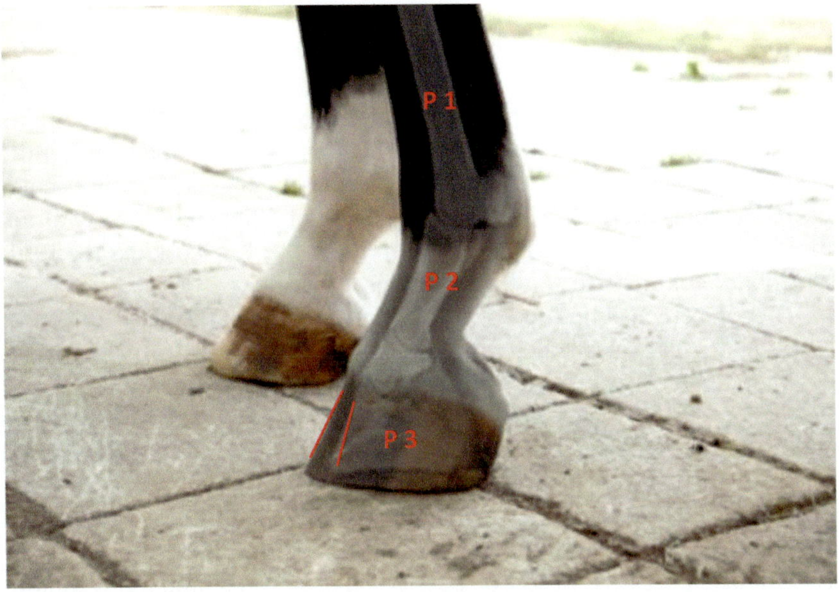

Figure 4.6 P1: Proximal phalanx. P2: Middle phalanx. P3: Distal phalanx (coffin/pedal bone). Laminitis in horses involves the rotation of the third phalanx (P3).

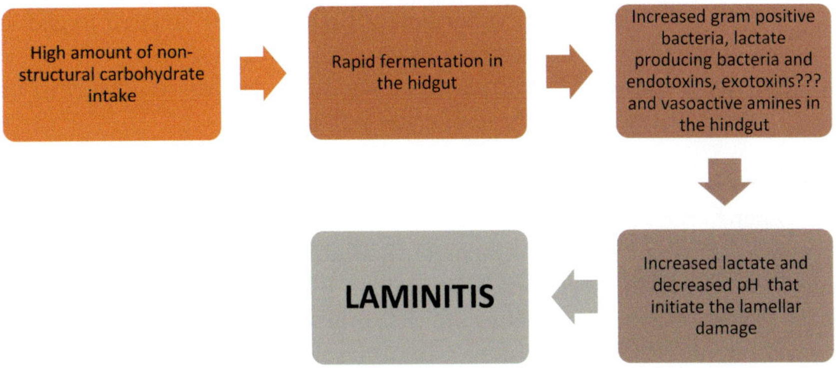

Figure 4.7 Basic schematic overview development of laminitis after consumption of high non-structural carbohydrate feeds (Garner et al., 1977).

- **Insulin-induced laminitis:** This model focuses on studying the role of insulin dysregulation in laminitis development. Horses or ponies with insulin dysregulation or other metabolic conditions associated with laminitis are given carbohydrates that elevate insulin levels or insulin injections to induce laminitis-like symptoms. This model helps researchers understand the mechanisms through which insulin dysregulation can contribute to hyperinsulinemia-associated laminitis (HAL).

Causes of laminitis

- **Breed predisposition:** Epidemiological research has identified endocrinopathic laminitis, characterized by equine metabolic syndrome (EMS) with insulin dysregulation (ID) and potentially pituitary pars intermedia dysfunction (PPID), as the predominant type of naturally occurring laminitis. Studies indicate that ponies and smaller, cold-blood horse breeds are at a heightened risk of developing this condition (Carslake et al., 2021; Donaldson et al., 2004; Karikoski et al., 2011; Pollard et al., 2019).
- **Diet:** Overconsumption of grain, high starch intake, lush grass, or a sudden change in diet can lead to laminitis. Pasture turnout with high non-structural carbohydrate content (simple sugars, fructans, and starch) can be a trigger factor for laminitis, even in lean, non-obese animals that do not have ID or increased basal plasma insulin concentrations.
- **Endocrine disorders:** Horses with conditions like EMS or PPID are at increased risk of laminitis (Bailey et al., 2008; Johnson, 2002).
- **Obesity:** Excessive weight or obesity can lead to ID, and a pro-inflammatory state puts additional stress on the hooves.
- **Trauma:** Severe trauma or excessive concussion on the hooves can trigger laminitis. Laminitis resulting from trauma is typically referred to as "supporting limb laminitis" when it occurs in the opposite limb due to lameness or injury in the other limb. "Road founder" related to excessive concussion is another type of trauma-related laminitis.
- **Systemic illnesses:** Certain illnesses like colic, septicemia, pleuritis, or retained placenta in mares can result in laminitis.

Laminitis is a multifactorial condition, and obesity is a major risk factor, but other factors such as diet, endocrine disorders, and systemic illnesses can also contribute to its development. A study (Wylie et al., 2013) investigated the association between body weight, BCS, and age with the prevalence of laminitis in horses. It found that overweight and obese horses and ponies had a significantly higher risk of developing laminitis than horses with a normal body weight and body condition. The study highlights the importance of managing weight and body condition to prevent laminitis in horses.

Another study (Nourian et al., 2009) investigated the role of trauma and exaggerated glucose-insulin response in the development of laminitis. Insulin's mitogenic pathway may contribute to lamellar proliferation. Abnormal lamellar mitosis can lengthen and weaken the lamellar, distal phalanx attachment apparatus, contributing to the clinical signs that appear. The researchers induced lameness in ponies by subjecting them to an exaggerated glucose-insulin response to feeding, which simulated the metabolic and endocrine conditions associated with laminitis. The study found that laminitis-like changes, including ultrastructural lesions, were observed in ponies' hooves after the induction of lameness. This suggests that trauma and the associated metabolic changes can contribute to the development of laminitis. Recent research has found that ID horses have different non-structural carbohydrate (NSC) thresholds to non-ID horses, and in ID horses and ponies, intakes above 0.1g/kg BW/meal lead to exaggerated insulin responses, which carry risks of HAL (Macon et al., 2022, 2023). This work shows the importance of restricted small meals in feeding the ID horses, as this equates to only 0.5 kg of a 10% NSC hay fed to a 500-kg horse. Research on the impact of feeds on non-ID horses can't be extrapolated to ID horses.

Symptoms: Symptoms of laminitis include lameness, pain, increased digital pulse, heat in hooves, reluctance to move, hesitance to walk or move and maybe adopting a "founder stance" to relieve pressure on the affected hooves, and increased lying down.

Phases: Laminitis in horses can be categorized into acute and chronic phases based on the progression and duration of the condition. The phases of laminitis include:

- **Acute phase:** The acute phase of laminitis is the initial stage and is characterized by the sudden onset of clinical signs. The common signs include lameness, increased digital pulse, heat in the hooves, reluctance to move, increased lying down, and a characteristic "founder stance" where the horse shifts their weight onto the hind limbs to relieve pressure on the front hooves. During this phase, there may be damage to the sensitive laminae, causing separation between the hoof wall and the coffin/pedal bone.
- **Subacute phase:** The subacute phase follows the acute phase and is characterized by a decrease in the severity of clinical signs. The horse may show reduced pain and inflammation, and the lameness may improve slightly. However, there can still be ongoing damage and inflammation within the hooves.
- **Chronic phase:** This phase occurs when the laminitis becomes long-term or recurring. Chronic laminitis can lead to permanent changes, such as rotation or sinking of the pedal bone, abnormal hoof growth, and the development of hoof wall distortions. Horses in the chronic phase may have ongoing lameness and require consistent management and specialized hoof care to alleviate discomfort.

Treatment/management of laminitis: Laminitis requires immediate veterinary attention. The treatment and management of laminitis can vary depending on the severity and underlying cause, but some common approaches include:

- **Pain management:** Ice boots are great for treating feet because the horse can stand in the boot filled with iced water, but a tub of iced water will work as well.
- **Hoof care:** Trimming the hooves to relieve pressure and realign the pedal bone–hoof wall axis is crucial after the acute stage. In some cases, supportive devices like therapeutic shoes or boots may be used (Figure 4.8).
- **Diet management:** Restricting access to high-sugar and high-starch foods is vital. Horses require a low-NSC, high-fiber diet. Forage should be less than 10%–12% NSC. However, forage alone will have deficiencies in key amino acids, minerals, and vitamins important for hoof health and repair, so a low-NSC and low-energy balancer pellet supplement is needed. As low-energy forage is often low in protein, the balancer should supply protein and amino acids, but very high levels/intakes of protein and amino acids in the balancer pellet should be avoided if the horse is ID (Loos et al., 2019). For extra hoof growth, a biotin, zinc, and methionine hoof supplement will be useful. If the affected horse is insulin dysregulated, supplements of chromium, fish oil, and psyllium have been shown to reduce hyperinsulinemia. Affected or at-risk horses should have no molasses, no treats, and no pasture access if ID.
- **Exercise management:** In the early stages, an affected horse or pony should be in a well-bedded stable or on sand. Controlled exercise and turnout on soft surfaces can help promote circulation and hoof health. In cases of severe laminitis, veterinarians will advise horses to be confined to stalls for an extended period of time.
- **Medications:** If an underlying hormonal disorder is present, medications to manage those conditions may be prescribed. NSAIDs may be prescribed to reduce pain and inflammation. Ertugliflozin may effectively reduce insulin concentrations in horses with EMS, and its use may hasten recovery from HAL (Sundra et al., 2023).
- **Weight loss:** through a combination of diet management and exercise, weight loss is a vital aim in ID most horses.
- **Monitoring:** Regular veterinary check-ups and radiographs (X-rays) may be needed to monitor the progress of treatment.

Maintaining a balanced diet, managing weight, and providing regular hoof care are all important in preventing laminitis.

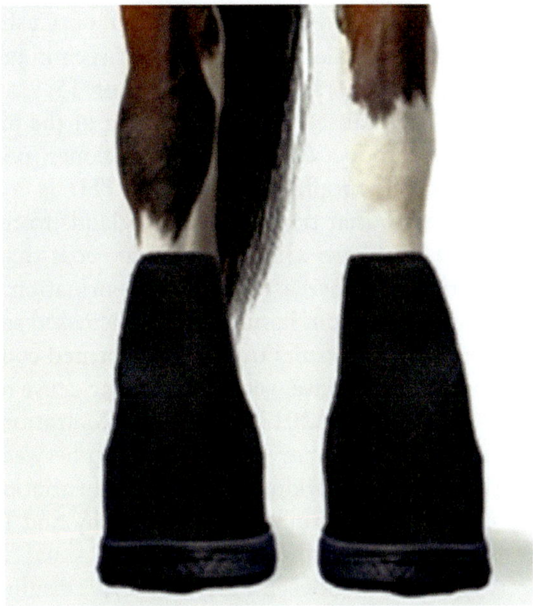

Figure 4.8 The image shows a horse's legs with an iced bandage.

4.6 The role of nutrition in endocrine diseases

Endocrine diseases in horses refer to a group of conditions that affect the normal metabolic processes within a horse's body. These disorders can result in abnormal functioning of various organ systems and can have significant health implications for the horse. Here are a few common metabolic disorders seen in horses:

- **Equine metabolic syndrome (EMS):** EMS has emerged as a major concern in modern veterinary medicine. EMS is linked to an increased risk of HAL. Evaluating genetic and metabolic predispositions to EMS in ponies involves evaluating episodes of laminitis in a herd kept on pasture, and ponies are twice as likely as other horse breeds to develop pasture-associated laminitis (Carter et al., 2009b; Menzies-Gow et al., 2010). ID is a constant feature of EMS, and increased generalized or regional adiposity is common. EMS is caused by a combination of genetic and environmental factors, particularly diets high in non-structural carbohydrates. ID is the central endocrine disorder of EMS. It is typically associated with increased generalized or regional adiposity (obese EMS), but it can also be detected in lean horses (not-obese EMS). The clinical presentation of EMS in horses includes obesity or local fat deposition, bilateral lameness or laminitis, and the occurrence of ID, which disrupts the homeostasis within insulin, glucose, and lipid metabolism (Stefaniuk-Szmukier et al., 2023).

- **Pituitary pars intermedia dysfunction (PPID) or Cushing's Disease:** PPID is an endocrine disorder most commonly seen in geriatric horses, affecting 20%–25% of horses over the age of 15 years (Ireland & McGowan, 2018). It is caused by a dysfunction of the pituitary gland, leading to excessive production of certain hormones, particularly cortisol. The adrenocorticotropic hormone (ACTH) is a hormone the pituitary gland releases that triggers adrenal glands to release cortisol. Horses with PPID may have a long, curly hair coat that fails to shed properly (hypertrichosis), increased thirst and urination, muscle wasting, abnormal fat distribution, laminitis, and increased susceptibility to infections. Hypertrichosis results from an augmented count of hair follicles in the active growth phase, yet its underlying cause remains poorly comprehended (Innerå et al., 2013). ACTH concentrations can be used to diagnose PPID, but there may be some overlap between normal and PPID populations due to individual and temporal variations. As ACTH concentrations rise in the autumn in both healthy and PPID animals, ACTH testing for PPID diagnosis necessitates seasonal adjustments. A link has been established between PPID and hyperinsulinemia in some affected horses and ponies, which has the potential to result in laminitis (Tadros et al., 2019). The management of the PPID is different in the ID horse compared to the non-ID horse. Seek advice from an equine nutritionist or a veterinarian with a special interest in nutrition.

The role of starch and sugar in nutrition-related disorders

High-NSC (non-structural carbohydrates) diets, commonly referred to as starch, have been associated with various digestive and metabolic disorders in horses, including colic, laminitis (Durham, 2009; Hudson et al., 2001), hindgut acidosis (Stewart et al., 2017), developmental orthopedic disease, PPID, equine gastric ulcer syndrome (Luthersson et al., 2009), and obesity (Hoffman, 2009). Increased behavioral and physiological reactivity, leading to nervousness or tension, has also been linked to high-starch diets, likely through microbiota changes (Bulmer et al., 2015; Bulmer et al., 2019). Muscular disorders such as exertional rhabdomyolysis and polysaccharide storage myopathy, resulting from excessive glycogen storage in muscles, are additional concerns associated with high starch and sugar intake (MacLeay, Sorum, et al., 1999; Valberg et al., 1999).

When high-starch diets reach the hindgut, microbiome alterations occur, increasing lactic acid production and causing a drop in pH, leading to acidosis (Geor & Harris, 2007; Merritt & Julliand, 2013). Lowering the pH in the large intestine also reduces fiber-degrading bacteria, impacting fiber digestion and the production of volatile fatty acids, leading to decreased slow-release energy production (Drogoul et al., 2001; Medina et al., 2002). Considering these factors, horse owners are advised to take into account the NSC or starch content when deciding on suitable concentrate feeds for their horses.

Nutrition plays a crucial role in the development, management, and prevention of equine metabolic disorders. The right diet can help regulate insulin levels, maintain a healthy body weight, and support overall metabolic health in horses. The key considerations regarding treatment and preventing nutrition and equine metabolic disorders are:

- **Weight management:** Obesity is a common cause of most metabolic disorders. Monitoring the horse's body condition score is critical for weight management. It is critical to monitor the horse's calorie intake and ensure that it corresponds to their energy requirements. Reducing calorie intake and increasing physical activity are critical for losing weight and improving insulin sensitivity (Durham et al., 2019; Kienzle & Bockhorni, 2018). Weighing the amount of forage and feed enables a precise understanding of what a horse consumes, allowing for the avoidance of unnecessary calories. Analyzing forage provides insights into the exact calorie and protein intake of the horse. Additionally, soaking hay can further decrease calorie content (Bochnia et al., 2021), and there's the option to minimize or eliminate concentrate feed intake altogether. Remember, a forage-only diet will need some supplementary protein, minerals, and vitamins. Achieving weight loss in a horse is possible by implementing a diet consisting of a measured weight of 50% hay and 50% barley straw (Dosi et al., 2020).
- **Carbohydrate restrictions:** Horses with metabolic disorders often benefit from avoiding feed high in NSC content from sugars and starches (Galinelli et al., 2021). These carbohydrates can contribute to hyperinsulinemia, ID, and weight gain, all of which lead to EMS. Limiting access to lush pastures, which tend to be high in sugars and calories, is critical for horses. Additionally, commercial feeds formulated specifically for horses with metabolic issues are available and can provide balanced nutrition while controlling carbohydrate intake. Good-quality forage, such as grass hay or low-sugar hay, should be the foundation of the horse's diet, but high-energy forages, which can contribute to obesity or failure to lose weight, should be avoided. Low-NSC forages are necessary for horses with metabolic disorders; both sugars and starches can cause insulin spikes. Soaking hay is another method for reducing NSC content (Bochnia et al., 2021). The NSC content of forage can be tested to ensure that it is suitable for horses with metabolic issues.
- **Number of meals and meal size:** For horses with metabolic disorders, feeding smaller meals more frequently throughout the day is essential (Kienzle & Bockhorni, 2018), as this avoids exceeding NSC intake thresholds (Macon et al., 2023). Double small-hole haynets or two haynets above each other also effectively slow hay intake and stretch limited hay over the day (Figure 4.9). This approach helps prevent

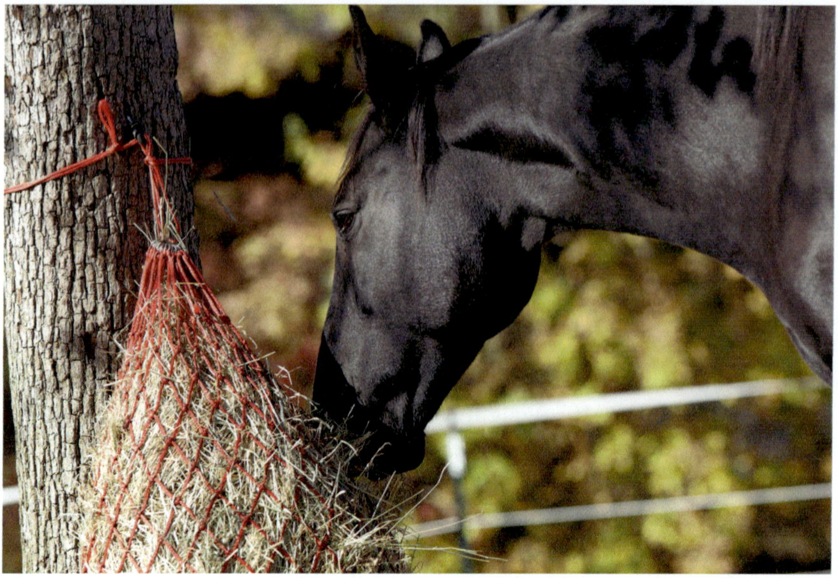

Figure 4.9 Horse eating hay from a haynet, which slows hay intake.

spikes in insulin levels associated with large meals and supports a more consistent metabolic response.

- **Balanced diet:** Providing a balanced diet is essential for horses with metabolic disorders. The diet should contain appropriate levels of energy, protein, vitamins, minerals, and essential fatty acids. It is important to avoid overfeeding or underfeeding, as both can have negative effects on the horse's metabolism. Low-energy balancer pellets with daily intakes ranging from 100 g to 1 kg, depending on the horse's requirements and BW, are vital to supplement nutrients deficient in forage-only diets.

Regular veterinary check-ups and monitoring are crucial for maintaining the health and well-being of horses with metabolic disorders.

4.7 The role of nutrition in myopathies

Myopathies in horses refer to a group of muscular disorders or diseases that can affect the muscles of horses. There are several types of myopathies that can affect horses; the most common types are:

- **Exertional rhabdomyolysis (ER):** ER is a condition that causes muscle cramping and damage during or after exercise. ER is influenced by both environmental factors and a genetic predisposition, with the highest occurrence rates reported among young, excitable female horses undergoing race training while on high-starch diets (MacLeay et al., 1999; MacLeay, Sorum, et al., 1999; MacLeay, Valberg, et al., 1999a). It is estimated to affect 5% of all thoroughbred racehorses in the US and UK and is the most common muscle disease affecting this breed (MacLeay, Sorum, et al., 1999; McGowan et al., 2002). It is thought to be related to a dysfunction in calcium regulation within muscle cells (Lentz et al., 1999). The condition may be inherited in an autosomal dominant manner with variable expression in thoroughbreds, meaning that recurrent exertional rhabdomyolysis (RER) could be a breed-specific genetic defect (MacLeay, Valberg, et al., 1999b). The symptoms of RER can range from mild to severe. They may include stiffness and reluctance to move, muscle pain or sensitivity to touch, sweating, trembling, or muscle fasciculations (twitching), dark or discolored urine due to the release of muscle proteins (myoglobin), abnormal gait or lameness, and swollen or firm muscles following mild to moderate exercise.

- **Polysaccharide storage myopathy (PSSM):** PSSM is a genetic muscle disorder characterized by abnormal storage of glycogen (a storage form of glucose) within skeletal muscle fibers. It predominantly affects draft breeds, warmbloods, and some Quarter Horses. Symptoms may include muscle stiffness, weakness, exercise intolerance, muscle damage, acute muscle atrophy, and gait abnormalities (Firshman et al., 2003). Type 1 PSSM can be diagnosed by genetic testing, but type 2 requires a muscle biopsy.
  - PSSM1 is a muscular disorder characterized by an anomalous buildup of glycogen in muscle cells due to a genetic mutation in a specific gene known as glycogen synthase 1 (GYS1). This condition is observed in various breeds, such as Quarter Horses, Paint Horses, and several draft horse breeds (Valberg et al., 1999).
  - PSSM2 encompasses a range of muscle disorders that also involve abnormal glycogen accumulation in muscle cells (Valberg et al., 2023). However, horses with PSSM2 do not possess the genetic mutation, and neither this disorder nor MFM can be diagnosed by genetic testing (Valberg et al., 2021).
- **Myofibrillar myopathy (MFM)** is a newly discovered disorder affecting Arabian and warmblood horses characterized by breaks in muscle fibers. It requires a biopsy for diagnosis. Warmbloods show exercise intolerance, with "reluctance to go forward or collect" being common signs, while Arabian horses have moderate tying-up episodes and have very high muscle enzyme levels (Valberg, 2021).

Management strategies for horses with PSSM or RER

- Providing a forage-based diet provides a consistent source of energy and helps maintain gut health. It is recommended to use grass hay rather than haylage. Avoid high-sugar, high-legume pastures. Super fibers such as beet pulp or soybean hulls are good high-energy sources for horses prone to tying up as well.

- Limit the starch and sugar intake by decreasing the intake of grains, sweet feeds, and high-sugar treats. The percentage of the total ration DE from NSC should be <15% for PSSM, and <20% for RER management (Geor et al., 2013; Pagan & Valberg, 2020).
- Adding fat to the diet such as vegetable oils can be beneficial to provide energy for horses prone to RER. Adding oil at a rate of >1 mL/kg BW, with the percentage of the total ration DE coming from fat being 20%–25%, is ideal (Geor et al., 2013; Pagan & Valberg, 2020). High-oil feeds such as stabilized rice bran can be used, and there are a number of low-NSC, high-fat, and high-fiber feeds for tying up, although only one feed is validated by research (McKenzie, 2003; Ribeiro et al., 2004).
- Horses with MFM need a moderate NSC and protein concentrate; supplementary amino acids and high fat content should be avoided (Valberg S.J., 2021).
- Provide an appropriate electrolyte supplement, especially during periods of increased sweating or intense exercise, to help maintain proper electrolyte balance.
- Adequate levels of vitamin E and selenium are important for muscle health. In regions with selenium-deficient soils, supplementation may be necessary.

4.8 The role of nutrition in asthma

Equine asthma covers the diseases formerly known as inflammatory airway disease (IAD) and heaves or recurrent airway obstruction (RAO). It is a chronic respiratory condition that affects horses, is similar to human asthma, and is characterized by the narrowing of the airways, increased mucus production, and inflammation in the lungs. Asthma is commonly seen in both younger (IAD) and middle-aged to older (RAO) horses, and is typically associated with an allergic or hypersensitivity reaction to certain environmental triggers such as airborne molds and particulate material (Couetil et al., 2020). The signs of asthma include persistent coughing, especially after exercise or exposure to dusty environments, labored breathing, nasal discharge, exercise intolerance, and wheezing (Figure 4.10).

The common causes include exposure to dusty or moldy environments, such as poorly ventilated stables or moldy hay, pollens, and allergens, poor air quality, such as with stalled horses or those kept in areas with poor air circulation may be exposed to high levels of ammonia, dust, and other respiratory irritants. There is a possibility that equine asthma has a genetic component. Environmental management and nutritional support are important aspects of asthma management, as shown in Table 4.3.

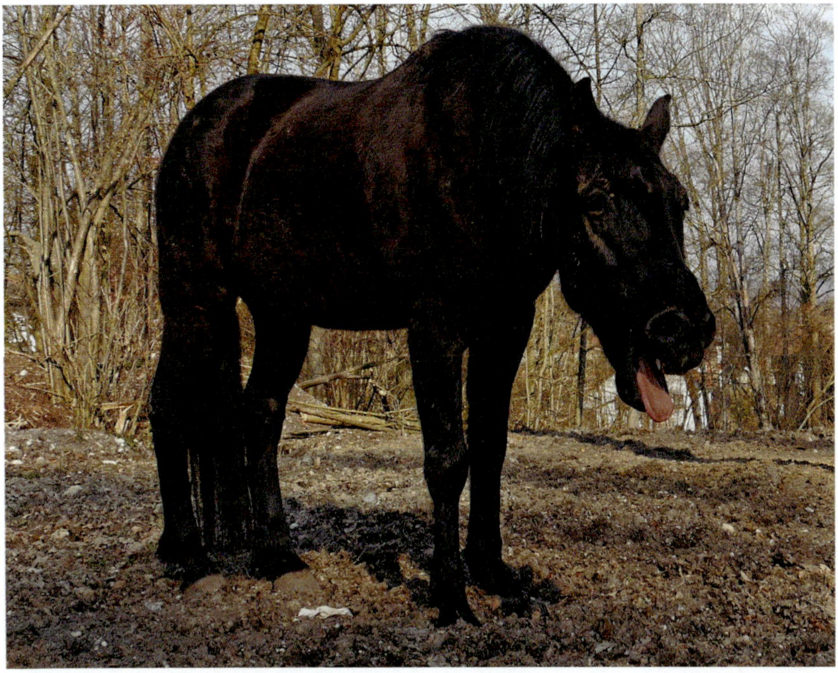

Figure 4.10 The illustration presents a horse coughing.

Table 4.3 Environmental management and nutritional support are important aspects of managing asthma

Environmental management	*Nutritional support*
▪ Provide a well-ventilated stable or living area for the horse. Good airflow helps reduce the concentration of dust, allergens, and respiratory irritants.	▪ Feed high-quality hay that has low dust content. Dusty hay can be a significant trigger for asthma. Consider alternative forage options, like haylage or complete pelleted feeds to minimize dust exposure, or steamed hay, which have lower dust levels.
▪ Use low-dust bedding materials, such as dust-extracted straw, shavings, or pelleted bedding (Kwiatkowska-Stenzel et al., 2017). Regularly clean and remove soiled bedding to minimize dust and mold accumulation.	▪ Soaking hay for 20–30 minutes in water before feeding can help reduce dust and allergen levels (Müller et al., 2015). Drain off the water to remove excess dust, but avoid over-soaking to prevent nutrient loss and bacterial or fungal proliferation.
▪ Provide access to pasture turnout whenever possible, as fresh air and grazing can benefit horses with respiratory conditions. Ensure the pasture is free from excessive dust, mold, or pollen sources.	▪ Long-chain omega-3 fatty acid supplementation provides an additional benefit to a low-dust diet in the management of horses with chronic lower airway inflammatory disease (Nogradi et al., 2015).

References

Ahmadi, F., Mirshahi, A., Mohri, M., Sardari, K., & Sharifi, K. (2021). Osteochondrosis dissecans (OCD) in horses: Hormonal and biochemical study (19 cases). *Veterinary Research Forum: An International Quarterly Journal*, *12*(3), 325–331. https://doi.org/10.30466/vrf.2020.104046.2495

Archer, D. C., & Proudman, C. J. (2006). Epidemiological clues to preventing colic. *Veterinary Journal*, *172*, 29– 39. https://doi.org/10.1016/j.tvjl.2005.04.002

Bailey, S. R., Habershon-Butcher, J. L., Ransom, K. J., Elliott, J., & Menzies-Gow, N. J. (2008). Hypertension and insulin resistance in a mixed-breed population of ponies predisposed to laminitis. *American Journal of Veterinary Research*, *69*(1), 122–129. https://doi.org/10.2460/ajvr.69.1.122

Bezděková, B., Jahn, P., & Vyskočil, M. (2008). Gastric ulceration, appetite and feeding practices in standardbred racehorses in the Czech Republic. *Acta Veterinaria Brno*, *77*(4), 603–607. https://doi.org/10.2754/avb200877040603

Bochnia, M., Pietsch, C., Wensch-Dorendorf, M., Greef, M., & Zeyner, A. (2021). Effect of hay soaking duration on metabolizable energy, total and prececal digestible crude protein and amino acids, non-starch carbohydrates, macronutrients and trace elements. *Journal of Equine Veterinary Science*, *101*, 103452. https://doi.org/10.1016/j.jevs.2021.103452

Bowden, A., Boynova, P., Brennan, M. L., England, G. C. W., Mair, T. S., Furness, W. A., Freeman, S. L., & Burford, J. H. (2020). Retrospective case series to identify the most common conditions seen 'out-of-hours' by first-opinion equine veterinary practitioners. *Veterinary Record*, *187*(10), 404–404. https://doi.org/10.1136/vr.105880

Brooks, S. A., Makvandi-Nejad, S., Chu, E., Allen, J. J., Streeter, C., Gu, E., McCleery, B., Murphy, B. A., Bellone, R., & Sutter, N. B. (2010). Morphological variation in the horse: Defining complex traits of body size and shape. *Animal Genetics*, *41*(s2), 159–165. https://doi.org/10.1111/j.1365-2052.2010.02127.x

Bulmer, L., McBride, S., Williams, K., & Murray, J.-A. (2015). The effects of a high-starch or high-fibre diet on equine reactivity and handling behaviour. *Applied Animal Behaviour Science*, *165*, 95–102. https://doi.org/10.1016/j.applanim.2015.01.008

Bulmer, L. S., Murray, J.-A., Burns, N. M., Garber, A., Wemelsfelder, F., McEwan, N. R., & Hastie, P. M. (2019). High-starch diets alter equine faecal microbiota and increase behavioural reactivity. *Scientific Reports*, *9*(1), 18621. https://doi.org/10.1038/s41598-019-54039-8

Cargile, J. L., Burrow, J. A., Kim, I., Cohen, N. D., & Merritt, A. M. (2004). Effect of dietary corn oil supplementation on equine gastric fluid acid, sodium, and prostaglandin E2 content before and during pentagastrin infusion. *Journal of Veterinary Internal Medicine*, *18*(4), 545. https://doi.org/10.1892/0891-6640(2004)18<545:EODCOS>2.0.CO;2

Carslake, H. B., Pinchbeck, G. L., & McGowan, C. M. (2021). Equine metabolic syndrome in UK native ponies and cobs is highly prevalent with modifiable risk factors. *Equine Veterinary Journal*, *53*(5), 923–934. https://doi.org/10.1111/evj.13378

Carter, R. A., Geor, R. J., Burton Staniar, W., Cubitt, T. A., & Harris, P. A. (2009a). Apparent adiposity assessed by standardised scoring systems and morphometric measurements in horses and ponies. *The Veterinary Journal*, *179*(2), 204–210. https://doi.org/10.1016/j.tvjl.2008.02.029

Carter, R. A., Treiber, K. H., Geor, R. J., Douglass, L., & Harris, P. A. (2009b). Prediction of incipient pasture-associated laminitis from hyperinsulinaemia, hyperleptinaemia and generalised and localised obesity in a cohort of ponies. *Equine Veterinary Journal*, *41*(2), 171–178. https://doi.org/10.2746/042516408X342975

Coenen, M., Kienzle, E., Vervuert, I., & Zeyner, A. (2011). Recent German developments in the formulation of energy and nutrient requirements in horses and the resulting feeding recommendations. *Journal of Equine Veterinary Science*, *31*(5–6), 219–229. https://doi.org/10.1016/j.jevs.2011.03.204

Cohen, N. D., Gibbs, P. G., & Woods, A. M. (1999). Dietary and other management factors associated with colic in horses. *Journal of the American Veterinary Medical Association*, *215*(1), 53–60.

Cohen, N. D., Matejka, P. L., Honnas, C. M., & Hooper, R. N. (1995). Case-control study of the association between various management factors and development of colic in horses. Texas Equine Colic Study Group. *Journal of the American Veterinary Medical Association*, *206*(5), 667–673.

Couetil, L., Cardwell, J. M., Leguillette, R., Mazan, M., Richard, E., Bienzle, D., Bullone, M., Gerber, V., Ivester, K., Lavoie, J.-P., Martin, J., Moran, G., Niedźwiedź, A., Pusterla, N., & Swiderski, C. (2020). Equine asthma: Current understanding and future directions. *Frontiers in Veterinary Science*, *7*. https://doi.org/10.3389/fvets.2020.00450

D'Eath, R. B., Tolkamp, B. J., Kyriazakis, I., & Lawrence, A. B. (2009). 'Freedom from hunger' and preventing obesity: The animal welfare implications of reducing food quantity or quality. *Animal Behaviour*, *77*(2), 275–288. https://doi.org/10.1016/j.anbehav.2008.10.028

Dionne, R. M., Vrins, A., Doucet, M. Y., & Pare, J. (2003). Gastric ulcers in standardbred racehorses: Prevalence, lesion description, and risk factors. *Journal of Veterinary Internal Medicine*, *17*(2), 218–222. https://doi.org/10.1111/j.1939-1676.2003.tb02437.x

Donaldson, M. T., Jorgensen, A. J. R., & Beech, J. (2004). Evaluation of suspected pituitary pars intermedia dysfunction in horses with laminitis. *Journal of the American Veterinary Medical Association*, *224*(7), 1123–1127. https://doi.org/10.2460/javma.2004.224.1123

Dosi, M. C. M., Kirton, R., Hallsworth, S., Keen, J. A., & Morgan, R. A. (2020). Inducing weight loss in native ponies: Is straw a viable alternative to hay? *Veterinary Record*, *187*(8). https://doi.org/10.1136/vr.105793

Drogoul, C., de Fombelle, A., & Julliand, V. (2001). Feeding and microbial disorders in horses: 2: Effect of three hay:grain ratios on digesta passage rate and digestibility in ponies. *Journal of Equine Veterinary Science*, *21*(10), 487–491. https://doi.org/10.1016/S0737-0806(01)70211-0

Dukti, S. A., Perkins, S., Murphy, J., Barr, B., Boston, R., Southwood, L. L., & Bernard, W. (2010). Prevalence of gastric squamous ulceration in horses with abdominal pain. *Equine Veterinary Journal*, *38*(4), 347–349. https://doi.org/10.2746/042516406777749164

Durham, A. E. (2009). The role of nutrition in colic. *Veterinary Clinics of North America: Equine Practice*, *25*(1), 67–78. https://doi.org/10.1016/j.cveq.2008.11.003

Durham, A. E., Frank, N., McGowan, C. M., Menzies-Gow, N. J., Roelfsema, E., Vervuert, I., Feige, K., & Fey, K. (2019). ECEIM consensus statement on equine metabolic syndrome. *Journal of Veterinary Internal Medicine*, *33*(2), 335–349. https://doi.org/10.1111/jvim.15423

Eades, S. C. (2017). Experimental model of laminitis: Starch overload. In J. K. Bellknap & R. Geor (Eds.), *Equine laminitis* (pp. 54–58). Wiley Blackwell.

Field, J. R., & Jeffcott, L. B. (1989). Equine laminits — Another hypothesis for pathogenesis. *Medical Hypotheses*, *30*(3), 203–210. https://doi.org/10.1016/0306-9877(89)90062-5

Firshman, A. M., Valberg, S. J., Bender, J. B., & Finno, C. J. (2003). Epidemiologic characteristics and management of polysaccharide storage myopathy in Quarter Horses. *American Journal of Veterinary Research*, *64*(10), 1319–1327. https://doi.org/10.2460/ajvr.2003.64.1319

Franklin, S. H., Brazil, T. J., & Allen, K. J. (2008). Poor performance associated with equine gastric ulceration syndrome in four Thoroughbred racehorses. *Equine Veterinary Education*, *20*(3), 119–124. https://doi.org/10.2746/095777308X282363

Galinelli, N., Wambacq, W., Broeckx, B. J. G., & Hesta, M. (2021). High intake of sugars and starch, low number of meals and low roughage intake are associated with Equine Gastric Ulcer Syndrome in a Belgian cohort. *Journal of Animal Physiology and Animal Nutrition*, *105*(S2), 18–23. https://doi.org/10.1111/jpn.13215

Garner, H. E., Hutcheson, D. P., Coffman, J. R., Hahn, A. W., & Salem, C. (1977). Lactic acidosis: A factor associated with equine laminitis. *Journal of Animal Science*, *45*(5), 1037–1041. https://doi.org/10.2527/jas1977.4551037x

Geor, R., Harris, P., & Coenen, M. (2013). *Equine applied and clinical nutrition*. Elsevier Saunders.

Geor, R. J., & Harris, P. A. (2007). How to minimize gastrointestinal disease associated with carbohydrate nutrition in horses. *AAEP Proceedings*, 178–185.

Giles, S. L., Rands, S. A., Nicol, C. J., & Harris, P. A. (2014). Obesity prevalence and associated risk factors in outdoor living domestic horses and ponies. *PeerJ*, *2*, e299. https://doi.org/10.7717/peerj.299

Glunk, E. C., Pratt-Phillips, S. E., & Siciliano, P. D. (2013). Effect of restricted pasture access on pasture dry matter intake rate, dietary energy intake, and fecal pH in horses. *Journal of Equine Veterinary Science*, *33*(6), 421–426. https://doi.org/10.1016/j.jevs.2012.07.014

Goodson, J., Tyznik, W. J., Cline, J. H., & Dehority, B. A. (1988). Effects of an abrupt diet change from hay to concentrate on microbial numbers and physical environment in the cecum of the pony. *Applied and Environmental Microbiology*, *54*(8), 1946–1950. https://doi.org/10.1128/aem.54.8.1946-1950.1988

Gough, S., Hallowell, G., & Rendle, D. (2020). A study investigating the treatment of equine squamous gastric disease with long-acting injectable or oral omeprazole. *Veterinary Medicine and Science*, *6*(2), 235–241. https://doi.org/10.1002/vms3.220

Harker, I. J., Harris, P. A., & Barfoot, C. F. (2011). The body condition score of leisure horses competing at an unaffiliated championship in the UK. *Journal of Equine Veterinary Science*, *31*(5–6), 253–254. https://doi.org/10.1016/j.jevs.2011.03.058

Harris, P. A., Ellis, A. D., Fradinho, M. J., Jansson, A., Julliand, V., Luthersson, N., Santos, A. S., & Vervuert, I. (2017). Review: Feeding conserved forage to horses: Recent advances and recommendations. *Animal*, *11*(6), 958–967. https://doi.org/10.1017/S1751731116002469

Hillyer, M. H., Taylor, F. G. R., & French, N. P. (2001). A cross-sectional study of colic in horses on Thoroughbred training premises in the British Isles in 1997. *Equine Veterinary Journal*, *33*(4), 380–385. https://doi.org/10.2746/042516401776249499

Hoffman, R. M. (2009). Carbohydrate metabolism and metabolic disorders in horses. *Revista Brasileira de Zootecnia*, *38*(spe), 270–276. https://doi.org/10.1590/S1516-35982009001300027

Hudson, J. M., Cohen, N. D., Gibbs, P. G., & Thompson, J. A. (2001). Feeding practices associated with colic in horses. *Journal of the American Veterinary Medical Association*, *219*(10), 1419–1425. https://doi.org/10.2460/javma.2001.219.1419

Innerå, M., Petersen, A. D., Desjardins, D. R., Steficek, B. A., Rosser, E. J., & Schott, H. C. (2013). Comparison of hair follicle histology between horses with pituitary pars intermedia dysfunction and excessive hair growth and normal aged horses. *Veterinary Dermatology*, *24*(1), 212. https://doi.org/10.1111/j.1365-3164.2012.01080.x

Ireland, J. L., Clegg, P. D., McGowan, C. M., McKane, S. A., Chandler, K. J., & Pinchbeck, G. L. (2012). Disease prevalence in geriatric horses in the United Kingdom: Veterinary clinical assessment of 200 cases. *Equine Veterinary Journal*, *44*(1), 101–106. https://doi.org/10.1111/j.2042-3306.2010.00361.x

Ireland, J. L., & McGowan, C. M. (2018). Epidemiology of pituitary pars intermedia dysfunction: A systematic literature review of clinical presentation, disease prevalence and risk factors. *The Veterinary Journal*, *235*, 22–33. https://doi.org/10.1016/j.tvjl.2018.03.002

Jansson, A., Harris, P., Davey, S. L., Luthersson, N., Ragnarsson, S., & Ringmark, S. (2021). Straw as an alternative to grass forage in horses—Effects on post-prandial metabolic profile, energy intake, behaviour and gastric ulceration. *Animals*, *11*(8), 2197. https://doi.org/10.3390/ani11082197

Jansson, A., & Lindberg, J. E. (2012). A forage-only diet alters the metabolic response of horses in training. *Animal*, *6*(12), 1939–1946. https://doi.org/10.1017/S1751731112000948

Jensen, R. B., Austbø, D., & Tauson, A.-H. (2012). Feeding forage before or after oats affects caecum pH profiles of the horse. In *Forages and grazing in horse nutrition* (pp. 327–330). Wageningen Academic Publishers. https://doi.org/10.3920/978-90-8686-755-4_41

Jensen, R. B., Danielsen, S. H., & Tauson, A.-H. (2016). Body condition score, morphometric measurements and estimation of body weight in mature Icelandic horses in Denmark. *Acta Veterinaria Scandinavica*, *58*(S1), 59. https://doi.org/10.1186/s13028-016-0240-5

Johnson, P. J. (2002). The equine metabolic syndrome. *Veterinary Clinics of North America: Equine Practice*, *18*(2), 271–293. https://doi.org/10.1016/S0749-0739(02)00006-8

Jonsson, H., & Egenvall, A. (2010). Prevalence of gastric ulceration in Swedish Standardbreds in race training. *Equine Veterinary Journal*, *38*(3), 209–213. https://doi.org/10.2746/042516406776866390

Julliand, S., Buttet, M., Hermange, T., Hillon, P., & Julliand, V. (2023). Effect of diet composition on glandular gastric disease in horses. *Journal of Veterinary Internal Medicine*, *37*(4), 1528–1536. https://doi.org/10.1111/jvim.16747

Kaneene, J. B., Miller, R., Ross, W. A., Gallagher, K., Marteniuk, J., & Rook, J. (1997). Risk factors for colic in the Michigan (USA) equine population. *Preventive Veterinary Medicine*, *30*(1), 23–36. https://doi.org/10.1016/S0167-5877(96)01102-6

Karikoski, N. P., Horn, I., McGowan, T. W., & McGowan, C. M. (2011). The prevalence of endocrinopathic laminitis among horses presented for laminitis at a first-opinion/referral equine hospital. *Domestic Animal Endocrinology*, *41*(3), 111–117. https://doi.org/10.1016/j.domaniend.2011.05.004

Kaya, G., Sommerfeld-Stur, I., & Iben, C. (2009). Risk factors of colic in horses in Austria. *Journal of Animal Physiology and Animal Nutrition*, *93*(3), 339–349. https://doi.org/10.1111/j.1439-0396.2008.00874.x

Kaya-Karasu, G., Huntington, P. J., Iben, C., & Onmaz, A. C. (2016). *Poor performance associated with equine gastric ulcer in an Arabian racehorse*. https://api.semanticscholar.org/CorpusID:201919226

Kienzle, E., & Bockhorni, T. (2018). Ernährung von Pferden mit Equine Pituitary Pars Interme dia Dysfunction („Cushing-Syndrom“) unter Pergolidtherapie. *Tierärztliche Praxis Ausgabe G: Großtiere / Nutztiere*, *46*(4), 249–256. https://doi.org/10.15653/tpg-170574

Kronfeld, D. S., Meacham, T. N., & Donoghue, S. (1990). Dietary aspects of developmental orthopedic disease in young horses. *Veterinary Clinics of North America: Equine Practice*, *6*(2), 451–465. https://doi.org/10.1016/S0749-0739(17)30551-5

Kwiatkowska-Stenzel, A., Witkowska, D., Sowińska, J., & Stopyra, A. (2017). The effect of stable bedding materials on dust levels, microbial air contamination and equine respiratory health. *Research in Veterinary Science*, *115*, 523–529. https://doi.org/10.1016/j.rvsc.2017.09.022

Lamglait, B., Vandenbunder-Beltrame, M., Trunet, E., & Lemberger, K. (2017). Description of gastric ulcers and of their suspected, associated risk factors in deceased wild equids at the Réserve Africaine de Sigean, France (2010–2016). *Journal of Zoo and Wildlife Medicine*, *48*(3), 668–674. https://doi.org/10.1638/2016-0249.1

Lentz, L. R., Valberg, S. J., Balog, E. M., Mickelson, J. R., & Gallant, E. M. (1999). Abnormal regulation of muscle contraction in horses with recurrent exertional rhabdomyolysis. *American Journal of Veterinary Research*, *60*(8), 992–999.

Lepeule, J., Bareille, N., Robert, C., Ezanno, P., Valette, J. P., Jacquet, S., Blanchard, G., Denoix, J. M., & Seegers, H. (2009). Association of growth, feeding practices and exercise conditions with the prevalence of Developmental Orthopaedic Disease in limbs of French foals at weaning. *Preventive Veterinary Medicine*, *89*(3–4), 167–177. https://doi.org/10.1016/j.prevetmed.2009.02.018

Lo Feudo, C. M., Stucchi, L., Conturba, B., Stancari, G., Zucca, E., & Ferrucci, F. (2022). Equine gastric ulcer syndrome affects fitness parameters in poorly performing Standardbred racehorses. *Frontiers in Veterinary Science*, *9*. https://doi.org/10.3389/fvets.2022.1014619

Longland, A. C., Ince, J., & Harris, P. A. (2011). Estimation of pasture intake by ponies from liveweight change during six weeks at pasture. *Journal of Equine Veterinary Science*, *31*(5–6), 275–276. https://doi.org/10.1016/j.jevs.2011.03.095

Loos, C. M. M., Dorsch, S. C., Elzinga, S. E., Brewster-Barnes, T., Vanzant, E. S., Adams, A. A., & Urschel, K. L. (2019). A high protein meal affects plasma insulin concentrations and amino acid metabolism in horses with equine metabolic syndrome. *The Veterinary Journal*, *251*, 105341. https://doi.org/10.1016/j.tvjl.2019.105341

Luthersson, N., Nielsen, K. H., Harris, P., & Parkin, T. D. H. (2009). Risk factors associated with equine gastric ulceration syndrome (EGUS) in 201 horses in Denmark. *Equine Veterinary Journal*, *41*(7), 625–630. https://doi.org/10.2746/042516409X441929

MacLeay, J. M., Sorum, S. A., Valberg, S. J., Marsh, W. E., & Sorum, M. D. (1999). Epidemiologic analysis of factors influencing exertional rhabdomyolysis in Thoroughbreds. *American Journal of Veterinary Research*, *60*(12), 1562–1566.

MacLeay, J. M., Valberg, S. J., Pagan, J. D., De La Corte, F., Roberts, J., Billstrom, J., McGinnity, J., & Kaese, H. (1999). Effect of diet on Thoroughbred horses with recurrent exertional rhabdomyolysis performing a standardised exercise test. *Equine Veterinary Journal*, *31*(S30), 458–462. https://doi.org/10.1111/j.2042-3306.1999.tb05265.x

MacLeay, J. M., Valberg, S. J., Sorum, S. A., Sorum, M. D., Kassube, T., Santschi, E. M., Mickelson, J. R., & Geyer, C. J. (1999a). Heritability of recurrent exertional rhabdomyolysis in Thoroughbred racehorses. *American Journal of Veterinary Research*, *60*(2), 250–256.

MacLeay, J. M., Valberg, S. J., Sorum, S. A., Sorum, M. D., Kassube, T., Santschi, E. M., Mickelson, J. R., & Geyer, C. J. (1999b). Heritability of recurrent exertional rhabdomyolysis in Thoroughbred racehorses. *American Journal of Veterinary Research*, *60*(2), 250–256.

Macon, E. L., Harris, P., Bailey, S., Barker, V. D., & Adams, A. (2022). Postprandial insulin responses to various feedstuffs differ in insulin dysregulated horses compared with non-insulin dysregulated controls. *Equine Veterinary Journal*, *54*(3), 574–583. https://doi.org/10.1111/evj.13474

Macon, E. L., Harris, P., Bailey, S., Caldwell Barker, A., & Adams, A. (2023). Identifying possible thresholds for nonstructural carbohydrates in the insulin dysregulated horse. *Equine Veterinary Journal*, *55*(6), 1069–1077. https://doi.org/10.1111/evj.13910

Marlin, D. J., Williams, J., Pickles, K., & Sykes, B. (2019). Horse owner understanding of equine gastric ulcer syndrome (EGUS). *Journal of Equine Veterinary Science*, *76*, 55. https://doi.org/10.1016/j.jevs.2019.03.049

McGowan, C. M., Fordham, T., & Christley, R. M. (2002). Incidence and risk factors for exertional rhabdomyolysis in thoroughbred racehorses in the United Kingdom. *Veterinary Record*, *151*(21), 623–626. https://doi.org/10.1136/vr.151.21.623

McKenzie, E. (2003). Nutritional management of exertional rhabdomyolysis. In *Current therapy in equine medicine* (pp. 727–734). Elsevier. https://doi.org/10.1016/B978-0-7216-9540-2.50197-3

Medina, B., Girard, I. D., Jacotot, E., & Julliand, V. (2002). Effect of a preparation of on microbial profiles and fermentation patterns in the large intestine of horses fed a high fiber or a high starch diet. *Journal of Animal Science*, *80*(10), 2600. https://doi.org/10.2527/2002.80102600x

Menzies-Gow, N. J., Katz, L. M., Barker, K. J., Elliott, J., De Brauwere, M. N., Jarvis, N., Marr, C. M., & Pfeiffer, D. U. (2010). Epidemiological study of pasture-associated laminitis and concurrent risk factors in the South of England. *Veterinary Record*, *167*(18), 690–694. https://doi.org/10.1136/vr.c5177

Merritt, A. M., & Julliand, V. (2013). Gastrointestinal physiology. In *Equine applied and clinical nutrition* (pp. 3–32). Elsevier. https://doi.org/10.1016/B978-0-7020-3422-0.00001-8

Müller, C. E., Nostell, K., & Bröjer, J. (2015). Microbial counts in forages for horses—Effect of storage time and of water soaking before feeding. *Journal of Equine Veterinary Science*, *35*(7), 622–627. https://doi.org/10.1016/j.jevs.2015.06.005

Nieto, J. E., Snyder, J. R., Vatistas, N. J., & Jones, J. H. (2009). Effect of gastric ulceration on physiologic responses to exercise in horses. *American Journal of Veterinary Research*, *70*(6), 787–795. https://doi.org/10.2460/ajvr.70.6.787

Nogradi, N., Couetil, L. L., Messick, J., Stochelski, M. A., & Burgess, J. R. (2015). Omega-3 fatty acid supplementation provides an additional benefit to a low-dust diet in the management of horses with chronic lower airway inflammatory disease. *Journal of Veterinary Internal Medicine*, *29*(1), 299–306. https://doi.org/10.1111/jvim.12488

Nourian, A. R., Asplin, K. E., McGowan, C. M., Sillence, M. N., & Pollitt, C. C. (2009). Equine laminitis: Ultrastructural lesions detected in ponies following hyperinsulinaemia. *Equine Veterinary Journal*, *41*(7), 671–677. https://doi.org/10.2746/042516409X407648

Pagan, J. D. (2003). The role of nutrition in developmental orthopedic disease: Nutritional management. In *Diagnosis and management of lameness in the horse* (pp. 543–548). Elsevier. https://doi.org/10.1016/B978-0-7216-8342-3.50064-4

Pagan, J. D., Hauss, A. A., Pagan, E. C., Simons, J. L., & Waldridge, B. M. (2022). Long-chain polyunsaturated fatty acid supplementation increases levels in red blood cells and reduces the prevalence and severity of squamous gastric ulcers in exercised Thoroughbreds. *Journal of the American Veterinary Medical Association*, *260*(S3), S121–S128. https://doi.org/10.2460/javma.22.06.0275

Pagan, J. D., & Valberg, S. J. (2020). Feeding performance horses with myopathies. In Proceedings. *Am Assoc Equine Pract*, *66*, 66–74.

Philippeau, C., Faubladier, C., & Julliand, V. (2009). Is there an impact of feeding concentrate before or after forage on colonic pH and redox potential in horses? *Applied Equine Nutrition and Training: Equine Nutrition and Training Conference (ENUTRACO) 2009*, 203–208. https://doi.org/10.3920/978-90-8686-669-4

Pollard, D., Wylie, C. E., Newton, J. R., & Verheyen, K. L. P. (2019). Incidence and clinical signs of owner-reported equine laminitis in a cohort of horses and ponies in Great Britain. *Equine Veterinary Journal*, *51*(5), 587–594. https://doi.org/10.1111/evj.13059

Potter, S., Bamford, N., Harris, P., & Bailey, S. (2016). Prevalence of obesity and owners' perceptions of body condition in pleasure horses and ponies in south-eastern Australia. *Australian Veterinary Journal*, *94*(11), 427–432. https://doi.org/10.1111/avj.12506

Pratt-Phillips, S., & Munjizun, A. (2023). Impacts of adiposity on exercise performance in horses. *Animals*, *13*(4), 666. https://doi.org/10.3390/ani13040666

Reeves, M. J., Salman, M. D., & Smith, G. (1996). Risk factors for equine acute abdominal disease (colic): Results from a multi-center case-control study. *Preventive Veterinary Medicine*, *26*(3–4), 285–301. https://doi.org/10.1016/0167-5877(95)00551-X

Ribeiro, W. P., Valberg, S. J., Pagan, J. D., & Gustavsson, B. E. (2004). The effect of varying dietary starch and fat content on serum creatine kinase activity and substrate availability in equine polysaccharide storage myopathy. *Journal of Veterinary Internal Medicine*, *18*(6), 887. https://doi.org/10.1892/0891-6640(2004)18<887:TEOVDS>2.0.CO;2

Scantlebury, C. E., Archer, D. C., Proudman, C. J., & Pinchbeck, G. L. (2015). Management and horse-level risk factors for recurrent colic in the UKgeneral equine practice population. *Equine Veterinary Journal*, *47*(2), 202–206. https://doi.org/10.1111/evj.12276

Smyth, G. B., Gordon, B. J., & Allen, D. (1998). *Physiology of the gastrointestinal tract. A field guide to colic management in the horse: The practitioner's reference*. Veterinary Medicine Publishing Co., 29–58.

Sorrentino, V. L., Wickens, C. L., Warren, L. K., Knight, C. W., Goff, B. F., & Causey, R. C. (2019). Effect of short stem forage mixed with grain to promote mastication in horses. *Journal of Equine Veterinary Science*, *76*, 122. https://doi.org/10.1016/j.jevs.2019.03.192

Stefaniuk-Szmukier, M., Piórkowska, K., & Ropka-Molik, K. (2023). Equine metabolic syndrome: A complex disease influenced by multifactorial genetic factors. *Genes*, *14*(8), 1544. https://doi.org/10.3390/genes14081544

Stefanyk, O., & Slivinska, L. (2021). Prevalence of gastric ulcer syndrome in horses with different exercise intensity. *Scientific Messenger of LNU of Veterinary Medicine and Biotechnologies*, *23*(102), 72–77. https://doi.org/10.32718/nvlvet10211

Stephenson, H. M., Green, M. J., & Freeman, S. L. (2011). Prevalence of obesity in a population of horses in the UK. *Veterinary Record*, *168*(5), 131–131. https://doi.org/10.1136/vr.c6281

Stewart, A. S., Pratt-Phillips, S., & Gonzalez, L. M. (2017). Alterations in intestinal permeability: The role of the "Leaky Gut" in health and disease. *Journal of Equine Veterinary Science*, *52*, 10–22. https://doi.org/10.1016/j.jevs.2017.02.009

Sundra, T., Kelty, E., & Rendle, D. (2023). Preliminary observations on the use of ertugliflozin in the management of hyperinsulinaemia and laminitis in 51 horses: A case series. *Equine Veterinary Education*, *35*(6), 311–320. https://doi.org/10.1111/eve.13738

Sykes, B. W., Bowen, M., Habershon-Butcher, J. L., Green, M., & Hallowell, G. D. (2019). Management factors and clinical implications of glandular and squamous gastric disease in horses. *Journal of Veterinary Internal Medicine*, *33*(1), 233–240. https://doi.org/10.1111/jvim.15350

Sykes, B. W., Hewetson, M., Hepburn, R. J., Luthersson, N., & Tamzali, Y. (2015). European college of equine internal medicine consensus statement—Equine gastric ulcer syndrome in adult horses. *Journal of Veterinary Internal Medicine*, *29*(5), 1288–1299. https://doi.org/10.1111/jvim.13578

Tadros, E. M., Fowlie, J. G., Refsal, K. R., Marteniuk, J., & Schott, H. C. (2019). Association between hyperinsulinaemia and laminitis severity at the time of pituitary *pars intermedia* dysfunction diagnosis. *Equine Veterinary Journal*, *51*(1), 52–56. https://doi.org/10.1111/evj.12963

Tinker, M. K., White, N. A., Lessard, P., Thatcher, C. D., Pelzer, K. D., Davis, B., & Carmel, D. K. (1997a). Prospective study of equine colic incidence and mortality. *Equine Veterinary Journal*, *29*(6), 448–453. https://doi.org/10.1111/j.2042-3306.1997.tb03157.x

Tinker, M. K., White, N. A., Lessard, P., Thatcher, C. D., Pelzer, K. D., Davis, B., & Carmel, D. K. (1997b). Prospective study of equine colic risk factors. *Equine Veterinary Journal*, *29*(6), 454–458. https://doi.org/10.1111/j.2042-3306.1997.tb03158.x

Traub-Dargatz, J. L., Kopral, C. A., Seitzinger, A. H., Garber, L. P., Forde, K., & White, N. A. (2001). Estimate of the national incidence of and operation-level risk factors for colic among horses in the United States, spring 1998 to spring 1999. *Journal of the American Veterinary Medical Association*, *219*(1), 67–71. https://doi.org/10.2460/javma.2001.219.67

Valberg, S. J. (2021). Diagnosis and Management of Myofibrillar Myopathy in Warmblood Performance Horses. *Proc AAEP*, *67*, 66–74.

Valberg, S. J., Finno, C. J., Henry, M. L., Schott, M., Velez-Irizarry, D., Peng, S., McKenzie, E. C., & Petersen, J. L. (2021). Commercial genetic testing for type 2 polysaccharide storage myopathy and myofibrillar myopathy does not correspond to a histopathological diagnosis. *Equine Veterinary Journal*, *53*(4), 690–700. https://doi.org/10.1111/evj.13345

Valberg, S. J., Macleay, J. M., Billstrom, J. A., Hower-Moritz, M. A., & Mickelson, J. R. (1999). Skeletal muscle metabolic response to exercise in horses with 'tying-up' due to polysaccharide storage myopathy. *Equine Veterinary Journal*, *31*(1), 43–47. https://doi.org/10.1111/j.2042-3306.1999.tb03789.x

Valberg, S. J., Williams, Z. J., Finno, C. J., Schultz, A., Velez-Irizarry, D., Henry, M. L., Gardner, K., & Petersen, J. L. (2023). Type 2 polysaccharide storage myopathy in Quarter Horses is a novel glycogen storage disease causing exertional rhabdomyolysis. *Equine Veterinary Journal*, *55*(4), 618–631. https://doi.org/10.1111/evj.13876

Vokes, J., Lovett, A., & Sykes, B. (2023). Equine gastric ulcer syndrome: An update on current knowledge. *Animals*, *13*(7), 1261. https://doi.org/10.3390/ani13071261

Ward, S., Sykes, B. W., Brown, H., Bishop, A., & Penaluna, L. A. (2015). A comparison of the prevalence of gastric ulceration in feral and domesticated horses in the UK. *Equine Veterinary Education*, *27*(12), 655–657. https://doi.org/10.1111/eve.12491

Weiss, D. J., Evanson, O. A., Green, B. T., & Brown, D. R. (2000). In vitro evaluation of intraluminal factors that may alter intestinal permeability in ponies with carbohydrate-induced laminitis. *American Journal of Veterinary Research*, *61*(8), 858–861. https://doi.org/10.2460/ajvr.2000.61.858

Wylie, C. E., Collins, S. N., Verheyen, K. L. P., & Newton, J. R. (2013). Risk factors for equine laminitis: A case-control study conducted in veterinary-registered horses and ponies in Great Britain between 2009 and 2011. *The Veterinary Journal*, *198*(1), 57–69. https://doi.org/10.1016/j.tvjl.2013.08.028

Index

For Product Safety Concerns and Information please contact our EU representative GPSR@taylorandfrancis.com Taylor & Francis Verlag GmbH, Kaufingerstraße 24, 80331 München, Germany